P9-CFP-784

Until
I Say
Good-Bye

Until I Say Good-Bye

MY YEAR

OF

LIVING

WITH JOY

I Say

Good-Bye

Susan Spencer-Wendel
with Bret Witter

HARPER

NEW YORK · LONDON · TORONTO · SYDNEY

HARPER

"Lift Me Up." Words and music by Kate Voegele. Copyright ©
2009 Universal Music Corp. and Communikate Music. All rights
controlled and administered by Universal Music Corp. All rights
reserved. Used by permission. Reprinted by permission of Hal
Leonard Corporation.

"For Good." From the Broadway musical *Wicked*. Music and lyrics
by Stephen Schwartz. Copyright © 2003 by Grey Dog Music. All
rights reserved. Used by permission of Grey Dog Music (ASCAP).

A hardcover edition of this book was published in 2013 by Harper-
Collins Publishers.

UNTIL I SAY GOOD-BYE. Copyright © 2013, 2014 by Susan Spencer-
Wendel. All rights reserved. Printed in the United States of America. No part of this book may be used or reproduced in any manner
whatsoever without written permission except in the case of brief
quotations embodied in critical articles and reviews. For information address HarperCollins Publishers, 10 East 53rd Street, New
York, NY 10022.

HarperCollins books may be purchased for educational, business,
or sales promotional use. For information please e-mail the Special
Markets Department at SPsales@harpercollins.com.

First Harper paperback published 2014.

Designed by William Ruoto

Library of Congress Cataloging-in-Publication Data has been applied for.

ISBN 978-0-06-224147-4 (pbk.)

14 15 16 17 18   OV/RRD   10 9 8 7 6 5 4 3 2 1

For Stephanie
whom God divined my sister

HAPPY THE MAN

Happy the man, and happy he alone,
He who can call today his own:
He who, secure within, can say,
Tomorrow do thy worst, for I have lived today.
Be fair or foul or rain or shine
The joys I have possessed, in spite of fate, are mine.
Not Heaven itself upon the past has power,
But what has been, has been, and I have had my hour.

—JOHN DRYDEN

Contents

Until
I Say
Good-Bye

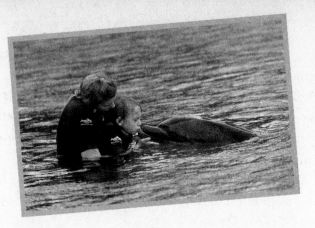

Introduction: Kissing the Dolphin

My son Wesley wanted to swim with the dolphins. He was turning nine on the ninth day of the ninth month—September 9, 2012—and this was his special request.

I had promised each of my three children a trip during the summer, each to a destination of their choice. A time for togetherness. A time to plant memories to blossom in their futures.

A present for them—and me.

In July, I traveled to New York City with Marina, my teenage daughter. In August, our family spent a week on Sanibel Island, off the west coast of Florida, at the request of my eleven-year-old son Aubrey.

The trips were part of a larger plan: a year I dedicated to living with joy. A year in which I took seven journeys with seven people central in my life. To the Yukon, Hungary, the Bahamas, Cyprus.

A year also of journeys inward: making scrapbooks from a

lifetime of photographs, writing, creating a haven in my own backyard—a Chickee hut with open sides, a palm frond roof, and comfy chairs where I summoned memories and friends.

Journeys I found more perfect in their doing than I had in their dreaming.

Wesley's trip was the simplest and the last. A three-hour drive in our minivan from our home in south Florida to Discovery Cove in Orlando.

"What a beautiful drive," my sister Stephanie commented, cheerful as ever, as we passed through the swampy monotony of central Florida.

Discovery Cove featured a huge artificial lagoon. A beach ringed one side, with rocks on the others. Palm trees rose above the lush landscape. Their fronds looked to me like fireworks heralding the occasion there.

We gathered on the beach in a drizzle, watching fins slice through the play area on the other side of the lagoon.

"Which one is ours?" Wesley asked. "Which one is ours?"

A trainer led us into the water. Suddenly a creature appeared before us: a smooth gray face with shining black eyes, a long mouth with edges turned upward as if in a smile. Her bottle-nose bobbed, signaling "I want to play!"

Wesley was over the moon. He jabbered and jumped, too excited to stand still. With his long blond hair, wetsuit, and blue eyes, he looked like the surfer boys I so admired in my youth.

Happy Birthday, my son.

Aubrey and Marina stood beside him, just as delighted.

"Isn't it mean to keep them penned up?" Marina asked no one in particular. Then the dolphin surfaced near her, and she made fun of her blowhole. Marina was near fifteen years old, her thoughts a jumble of the juvenile and the adult.

The trainer introduced us. Her name was Cindy—the dolphin, not the trainer. Cindy swam by slowly, allowing us to run our hands down her body. I was stunned by her size: eight and a half feet long, five hundred pounds of stone-solid muscle.

"What does she feel like?" the trainer asked.

"A Coach purse," wisecracked hubby John.

"I love Cindy!" Wesley gushed.

Cindy was more than forty years old. I asked if she had children.

"No, Cindy's a career woman," said the trainer.

Like me, a lifelong journalist. But I had children. I had the pleasure of standing with them in waist-deep water and feeling the skin of an aquatic wonder.

The trainer asked us to lift our hands to signal Cindy. Make a motion like you are reeling in a fishing line, and Cindy makes a sound just like it.

Wesley's mouth dropped open in amazement. "I love Cindy!" he said.

With the trainer's help, Wes grabbed her dorsal fin. He laid his body flat along her back, and for the next half hour Cindy pulled us one by one through the water. First the children, then Stephanie and John.

When it was my turn, I declined. "Let Wesley take my ride," I said. For this day was his day. The wonder on his face was obvious as Cindy skimmed him through the water.

We took many photos that day. Of Wesley. Of Aubrey and Marina. Of our family, smiling together on the beach in the rain.

There is one I adore: John holding me half out of the water, so that I might kiss Cindy on her smiling snout.

At the moment, I thought only of the gentle giant in front of me, of the smooth cool of her bottle-nose as I kissed it. A memory made.

When I saw the photo, I thought of the gentle giant behind me, lifting me as he does every day. I thought of my children, whose happiness enriches me. Of my sister and friends, who make me laugh.

I thought of Wesley, whose ninth birthday is likely the last I will share.

I cannot walk. I was rolled to the lagoon in a wheelchair.

I cannot support my own weight, even in water. John carried me from the chair and held me so I would not drown.

I cannot lift my arms to feed myself or hug my children. My muscles are dying, and they cannot return. I will never again be able to move my tongue enough to clearly say, "I love you."

Swiftly, surely, I am dying.

But I am alive today.

When I saw the photograph of myself kissing the dolphin, I did not cry. I was not bitter for what I had lost. I smiled instead, living the joy.

Then turned in my wheelchair, as best I could, and kissed John too.

Liftoff

July–September

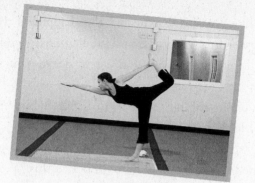

Still Lucky

It's odd to think of my autopilot life, the one before.

Forty-plus hours a week working a job I loved, writing about the local criminal courts for the *Palm Beach Post*. Another forty navigating the daily dance of sibling warfare, homework, and appointments—pediatrician, dentist, orthodontist, psychiatrist (no surprise, eh?).

Hours at music lessons with my children—or driving between them.

Evenings spent folding laundry on our dining room table.

An occasional dinner with friends or my sister Stephanie, who lived down the street.

A quiet float in the backyard pool with my husband, a few minutes at the end of the day, interrupted by a kiddie disagreement over television channels or six-year-old Wesley's out-of-nowhere request to draw on our spoons.

"Okay. On the white plastic ones. Not the silver ones!"

I felt lucky.

I felt happy.

And like anyone, I expected that happiness would sail on and on—through proms and graduations, weddings and grandchildren, retirement and a few decades of slow decline.

Then one night in the summer of 2009, while undressing for bed, I looked down at my left hand.

"Holy shit," I yelped.

I turned to my husband John. "Look at this."

I held up my left hand. It was scrawny and pale. In the palm, I could see the lines of tendons and the knobs of bones.

I held up my right hand. It was normal.

"You need to go to the doctor," John said.

"Okay."

I was too stunned to say anything else. It looked like my hand was dying. But I wasn't worried. All I thought was, How am I going to work this into my schedule?

I visited my family doctor, a kind woman who asked me five different ways if there was any pain in my left hand or arm.

"None," I answered.

"Well, it's probably not carpal tunnel then. I want you to see a neurologist."

And thus began a year-long odyssey of doctors' visits. Of attempts to explain my withered limb. To find an answer other than the one John, who had been researching on his own, mentioned at the end of my first neurologist appointment: ALS.

To which I replied: "What's that?"

ALS, more commonly known as Lou Gehrig's disease, is a neuromuscular disorder wherein nerves to muscles die, causing the muscles to die as well. It is progressive, meaning it always moves forward, from muscle to muscle. There is no known cause. No treatment. And no cure.

ALS would mean the death in my left hand would spread to my arm. Then through the rest of my body. I would weaken piece by piece, until I was paralyzed.

And then, usually within three to five years of the first symptoms, I would die.

No, that couldn't happen. No. There had to be another explanation.

Perhaps an injury? A few months before, I had fallen so hard while Rollerblading to my mother's house that the imprint of concrete remained on my left hand for an hour.

Sure enough, I had a bulging disk in my back . . . but not where it would affect my hand.

Dr. Jose Zuniga, my first neurologist, suggested Hirayama disease, a mysterious loss of muscle function disorder. The description fit my symptoms, except for one thing: most victims were Japanese.

"You're not Japanese," Dr. Zuniga observed.

I'll go with it, I thought. Went straight to the grocery store and bought sushi. Passed over the wussy California rolls and selected an eel roll instead.

It wasn't Hirayama disease.

An ALS specialist, Dr. Ram Ayyar, suggested multifocal neuropathy, a progressive muscle disorder that often begins in the hands. Unlike with ALS, there was a test for MFN. It cost $3,000. As I learned the hard way, my insurance wouldn't cover it. I was more upset and frustrated by that than by the test result: negative for multifocal neuropathy.

I saw four specialists in six months. I traveled to Cyprus, searching for a hereditary cause.

When nothing turned up, I stopped having tests. I entered a year of denial. I mean the sky-is-green kind of denial. One so obtuse and myopic, it's embarrassing now to admit to it.

When I started struggling with yoga in spring 2010, I had a friend take pictures of me in all twenty-six Bikram poses in the unlikely event I would be unable to continue.

At my parents' fiftieth anniversary celebration in November, John had to cut my prime rib. I could eat fine, but couldn't do the knife-and-fork tango anymore.

Too weak to carry my reporter's briefcase at work, I switched to a rolling bag. "I guess ya wanna look like the lawyers," said a reporter colleague.

I said not a word.

In January 2011, while brushing my teeth, I noticed my tongue twitching. No matter how much I tried, I couldn't stop it.

A few weeks later, I was having dinner at my sister Stephanie's house when I noticed her eyes widen. John was holding a fork, waiting to feed me. Wait, when had that become our routine?

"Stop it, John," I snapped. "I can feed myself."

For dessert, Steph served peanut butter pie. My tongue wasn't working. "Ya trying to kill me?" I joked, after giving up on moving the sticky wad around my mouth.

I refused to submit. Consciously, at least.

But we are creatures of the subconscious. I bought the book *Buddhism for Dummies*, trying to get a major Zen on and calm my mind.

I went for a long weekend to New Orleans with my best friend Nancy and our husbands. It was just after Mardi Gras 2011. So "just after," in fact, that the streets were still filled with streamers, beads, and garbage.

Nancy wanted to tour the Hurricane Katrina disaster zone. I begged off, more interested in distraction. One night on Bourbon Street, John and I found ourselves in front of a strip club.

Now, strip clubs are not my style. I had been to one just twice before in my life, both times as a newspaper reporter.

The first time, a patron was suing a stripper after she struck him in the face with her huge stripper shoe during her dance act. The man had a detached retina and broken orbital bone.

Really.

The second time I was on a story about a missing person whose relative worked at a place called the Kitten Club. I wandered in just as she was twirling all two hundred pounds of herself round the stage. Her breasts were like twins wrestling.

"Let's go in!" I said to John on Bourbon Street. "Let's really take our mind off things."

The place was packed. We musta looked like big spenders, because the bouncer sat us right at the edge of the stage.

The act consisted of three women—nude but for their four-inch plaid schoolgirl skirts—and a dirty-looking mattress.

One woman had recently given birth, her body tight except for her flabby, stretch-marked belly. She looked as if her milk had just come in. She tried and tried to get us to plant bills between those breasts.

"Come on, honey! Loosen up!" she said to me.

"For cryin' out loud," I said to John. "Just give her some cash for the baby and let's go."

We hunted down a less skanky place—one with a vast stage and club chairs. We sat waaaay back from the stage.

The women danced on poles. They pulled themselves up and down, straddled, curled, right side up, sideways, and upside down. They posed like leaping reindeer. Distractions galore, but I stared at their hands.

Holding.

Gripping.

Strong.

I looked down at my useless left hand, knowing that I could never grip like that again. My pole-dancing days were over before they began.

The next morning at breakfast with Nancy, I reported the bad fashion news from Bourbon Street: "Leg warmers are making a comeback."

We laughed, my hand forgotten.

Nancy and I always laugh when we're together.

But when we hugged good-bye at the airport, I saw the truth in Nancy's eyes. Concern. Sadness. She knew I had ALS. And so did I.

I started to cry, right there in the New Orleans airport.

"Don't cry," Nancy said. "Please don't cry."

She started imitating our octogenarian airport shuttle driver, who had talked loudly on his cell phone for ten minutes before saying, "Aw, wait, you're ma COU-SIN Willie!"

We laughed and parted, both drying our eyes.

Back home, I tumbled into depression.

I had held my fears at bay for more than a year. I had believed in my health, even as my weakness spread. I had immersed myself in motherhood, work, marriage, dear friends.

That spring, I began to do what I had warned myself against. Instead of living the moment, I slipped into dreading the future with ALS.

I thought of myself unable to walk and eat. Unable to hug my children and tell them I love them. I would sink into paralysis, my body incapacitated, but my mind untouched. I would understand and experience every loss. Then die with my children so young.

I began to dwell in that future. When I sat down for a meal, I thought about not being able to chew. I lay awake at night and stared at the ceiling, thinking, "One day, Susan, this is all you will be able to do. And it will happen soon."

What I feared most wasn't death. It was being entirely dependent on others. A burden on my family and the ones I loved.

I mentioned my fear that I had the disease to a brilliant lawyer friend. "Oh, ALS is worse than a death sentence," she quipped. I never spoke to her again.

For a long time, I never spoke of ALS, because I believed that too, that my future was worse than death.

I should end this now, I started thinking. With dignity, on my own terms.

I thought of suicide about as often as you see a butterfly. It would flutter into my mind, and I would study it, marveling at its symmetry. Then it would flit away, and I would forget, for it was only a passing thing.

Until it returned the next day, and the next. Because my

mind was a garden. Tended, cultivated, but unchecked on the edges. A perfect place for butterflies.

I thought of hiring a hit man. Go into a dark alley on the other side of town and be "murdered." I had sat in court with hit men many times. I was uniquely qualified for a premeditated murder—of myself.

But after a while, I let it go. Dumb idea. Messy. Awful.

I asked friends to help me. Then thought of how that would put them in jeopardy of being arrested. I changed my request: Come and read to me, please, when I can move no longer.

The butterfly returned, entrancing.

I ordered two books on suicide from the dozens listed on Amazon. I thought deeply about my personal belief that we as human beings should be able to choose how we die.

I found an organization in Switzerland called Dignitas, where the terminally ill die as they wish: Immediately. Peacefully. Legally.

Perfect.

Then I read this: "In order to access the service of an accompanied suicide, someone has to . . . possess a minimum level of physical mobility (sufficient to self-administer the drug)."

With ALS, I would lose the ability to raise a glass or even swallow its fatal cocktail. The esophagus, after all, is lined with muscles. It dies too.

I did not register for Dignitas.

I did not read the books.

Know those people who talk on and on about each headache? Who cannot sneeze without complaining?

I am not like those people.

I kept my mouth shut. I kept working. Raising my children. Living. Even John didn't know my thoughts. Until one day, while looking for stamps, he found the suicide books in my desk drawer.

"I glanced through them," I told him truthfully. "I thought about it. But I never formed a plan."

"Please, Susan . . ."

"I won't. I could never do that to you." I paused. "I could never do that to our children."

I do not think my death will ruin my family's lives. But I realize the way I die may affect their ability to live with delight. To live with joy.

A suicide would teach my children that I was weak.

When I am strong.

I made the neurologist appointment. June 22, 2011, four days after my son Aubrey's tenth birthday.

I had not been to the doctor in a year, and I was tired of putting it off. Tired of the tension of anticipating the two-by-four about to whack me in the head.

I spent the evening before the appointment in Miami, alone, for I did not want to talk. John granted my wish. Love is agreeing, even when you don't understand.

I stayed at my friend Nancy's brother's bachelor pad in Miami Beach. His unit was in an old open-air art deco building on the water. Second floor. I struggled to drag my overnight bag up the stairs.

He had left a key under his mat. I asked a neighbor to turn it in the lock for me.

The fridge was empty. A sheet covered the window. Pictures of his and Nancy's family topped antique furniture. I recalled seeing the furniture in their childhood home.

Nancy's brother, a filmmaker, had a trove of movies and books, including travel guides from around the world. I thought of my own extensive travels, of the friendship of those faces in the pictures.

I thought of the love I had known in my life. That most perfect, selfless kind felt nursing my child in the moonlight. That thrilling, romantic kind where all you want to do in the moonlight is please the other.

I am lucky, I thought. I have known remarkable love.

I am content no matter what happens tomorrow.

Nancy texted me: "Hear you're going to Miami. Thinking of you."

"Didn't wanna worry you," I replied.

I struggled to open the door to the apartment balcony. I sat outside and smoked, a habit that had become a comfort to me.

I practiced, among other things, being alone. Not a comfortable state for me. We are born alone and die alone, but all my favorite moments of life had been spent with someone else.

I thought of the victims and families I had seen in my ten years as a court journalist. I thought of how many had persevered through tragedy—and how others never recovered.

I psyched myself for my tragedy tomorrow.

I thought: When someone tells you that you have ALS, you have to steel yourself right away. No crying. No breaking down. You have to make a strong start.

I had learned this in competitive swimming, the coach drilling us on strong starts. Head tucked, ready to explode off the block.

Steady wins the race, right? That's what they always say. Steady wins.

Finally, I had enough of thinking. I picked the most jarring movie on the shelf: *Blow*. Cocaine! Violence! Distraction! Perfect! I took a sleeping pill and went to bed fully clothed.

In the morning, I took a cab to an unremarkable building in downtown Miami. People walked about in scrubs and stethoscopes, heads bent over their iPhones. I wondered which was the doctor who would change my life.

John arrived. Late, as always.

He'll be late to my funeral, I thought. That made me smile. Never change, John. Please never change.

In the office, a kind representative of MDA (the Muscular Dystrophy Association) circulated, greeting patients like old friends. A nurse took my vitals. My blood pressure was lower than normal—90 over 60. I breathed, slowly and deeply.

The nurse took us to an examining room.

Dr. Ashok Verma entered, a tall, distinguished Indian man with that disarming Anglo-Indian accent I like so much. Dr. Verma is the head of the University of Miami's ALS clinic.

He looked over my records.

He asked a few questions, did some strength testing, sat back at his desk, and chirped: "I believe you have ALS."

He sounded like he was inviting me to a birthday party. And he was smiling. I don't know if it was a caring smile or a nervous smile, but I will always remember that smile.

Now, I had planned how I would react when I heard those words. I had steeled myself. Strong. A burst off the starting block. An explosion of energy propelling me into the race.

I dropped my head for the start . . . and began to cry.

I could not stop, any more than I could stop my breathing or my heartbeat. I cried and cried.

Dr. Verma kept chirping about his ALS clinic, about how he wanted me to come there. "We have to stop pretending it's something else."

John was clearly annoyed. "Just hold on," he said. "Let's give her a minute."

I remember snot. Snot filling my nostrils, oozing out of them. I remember thinking how cruel a journalist colleague was when he had ridiculed a man testifying, weeping and dripping snot as he lamented killing six in a car accident.

So odd, eh? What the mind remembers when.

Dr. Verma held out a box of Kleenex. John wiped my face. I composed myself enough to talk, and pulled out my trump card.

Stem cells—my own personal stash.

Around the world, researchers were studying stem cells, trying to cure degenerative disease. I recalled the story of a local police officer with ALS whose buddies held fund-raisers to send him abroad for stem cell treatment.

And I had my own private stash, straight from the font of life. When my sons were born, I banked their umbilical cord blood, a treasure chest of cells to be used to fight future disease.

"Perhaps," I said, "there's a researcher who could use those stem cells on me?"

"The problem," Dr. Verma began slowly, "is that the researchers don't know how to get the stem cells to go to the right place."

He said he'd had forty-five ALS patients go abroad for stem cell treatment. None were cured or had their lives extended. All were left poorer. "In their pockets," Dr. Verma said, patting his.

I had long decided, come what may, I would not bankrupt my family chasing a cure. I would not clamor to be part of a clinic trial, only to receive a placebo. I would not doctor-hunt or go Google crazy, searching for someone to give me false hope.

That's that, I thought, as John wiped my nose once again.

We walked out in silence.

Drove in silence.

"I'm hungry," John said, confirming what I already well knew—the man can eat at any time.

We went to Burger King. I sat outside on a parking barrier, smoking a cigarette, while John went inside for food.

Now, I had watched Lou Gehrig's farewell speech of 1939 a number of times. The one where he declared himself the luckiest man on the face of the earth, even after "catching a bad break." Even after being diagnosed with a disease that would rob him of his talent, and then his life.

I had wondered if that was true. Did he really feel that way? Or was it a grand thought that only came to Gehrig surrounded by tens of thousands of applauding fans?

And then it came to me too, alone, seated on a parking barrier outside Burger King. No, not a muzzy moment, but my life in focus, tack sharp.

Forty-four years of perfect health. I had rarely even had a head cold or tooth cavity.

Forty-four years, and the sickest I had ever been was after I ate a bad chicken sandwich in South America.

I had three easy pregnancies, each producing a rosy, pudgy babe. Three breezy C-sections where I was walking the next day.

I had known abiding love; traveled the world; married a great partner; worked a job I adored.

I knew where I came from. Adopted as an infant by dutiful parents, I had met my birth mother at age forty and the family of my birth father soon after. I knew my ALS was not inherited from them. I knew my rosy, pudgy babes need not fear my fate.

I was alive. I had a year. Maybe more, but I knew I had one more year at least of good health.

I determined, right there in the Burger King parking lot, to spend it wisely.

To take the trips I'd longed to take and experience each pleasure I'd longed for as well.

To organize what I was leaving behind.

To plant a garden of memories for my family to bloom in their futures.

Lou Gehrig was an athlete. ALS took his talent immediately.

But I was a writer. ALS could curl my fingers and weaken my body, but it could not take my talent.

I had time to express myself. To build a place of my own with comfy chairs, where I could think and write and sit with friends. Where I could wander through my own garden of memories and write them down.

A wandering that became, beyond my every fantasy, this book.

A book not about illness and despair, but a record of my final wonderful year.

A gift to my children so they would understand who I was and learn the way to live after tragedy:

With joy.

And without fear.

If Lou Gehrig could feel lucky, then so could I.

So should I.

I tucked my head once again in the starting block, steeling myself for the race.

"I'm glad that's over," I told John when he returned with a coffee for me, a Whopper for himself. "And I still feel incredibly lucky."

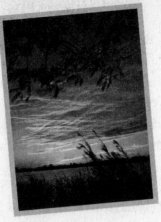

The Clinic

The clinic.

Ah, how I love that word.

Conjures notions of a kind nurse and a bed and a Popsicle and a chance to go home from school and sit and watch soap operas with Mom.

Dr. Verma's clinic, though, was the University of Miami's multidisciplinary comprehensive ALS clinic, located at St. Catherine's Rehabilitation Hospital in North Miami Beach. The name should have been my first clue.

John and I arrived about 1:00 p.m. Three hours after my appointment with Dr. Verma. Two hours after my diagnosis with ALS. An hour after I'd vowed to live with joy, while John wolfed down a Whopper.

The clinic was essentially a doctor's office. There was a waiting area with an admittance desk, doors, and those doctor mags. The patients looked normal. An older man and his wife. An older woman and her very, very pregnant daughter. We chatted about her coming child.

She asked if we had children.

For the first time that day, I saw John tear up.

Then the doors opened, and the medical staff streamed in to "begin clinic." Everyone seemed to be scurrying, including the woman at the center of it all, Ginna, a doctor of nursing. Dr. Nurse, I soon divined, was in charge of air traffic control.

She ushered us to an examining room. In walked the physical therapist, a petite woman in sensible shoes with a harness-looking thingy around her waist, as if she were going rappelling off a cliff.

Cheerfully, the therapist rattled off questions. "When were you diagnosed?"

"Today."

"Oh."

She did some strength testing. "Good," she said. "How do you feel?"

"Fine."

"You'll need physical therapy to keep you strong. When did the symptoms start?"

"Two years ago."

"That's wonderful! See you next time!"

Next came the respiratory therapist, who had me blow.

"Very good!" she proclaimed. "You're breathing well! We will monitor you for problems as your tongue and throat muscles weaken."

A half hour—*bing!*—and she was gone, just like the physical therapist before her. John and I looked at each other. We were in shock, reacting without understanding.

And then, *bing*, right on schedule, in came the speech pathologist.

Oh, I get it, I thought. It's speed dating. Dr. Nurse was the proctor, keeping the clinicians rotating on a fixed schedule.

Jeez, I wondered, how many people have this disease?

"I've had enough," I said. "I'm leaving."

"But you have more appointments!" Dr. Nurse protested.

"Not today."

She told me of a patient who had ALS for thirty years and still golfed at seventy. "Slow as your disease has progressed, you could end up like that," she said. "Maybe. We just don't know."

Maybe I have years. Maybe. But not because I attended this clinic. This was a cattle call, not treatment. *There is no cure for ALS!* my brain screamed. They were measuring my slide to death.

"See you next time," Dr. Nurse said, with a friendly smile.

I don't think so, I thought, as John escorted me out the door.

I would eventually find my own psychologist and physical therapist. But I would not be attending Dr. Verma's clinic.

I had been an official ALS patient for less than a day, and I already knew how I did not want to approach my disease.

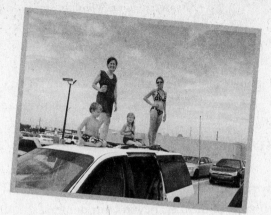

The Wonder

So what do you do when you don't want to study yourself? You look outward. Or more precisely, for me, you look up.

I have always been a lover of the heavens. To me, they are far more than a permanent ceiling. I look to the sky each day for glory—in a lavender sunset or brilliant moonrise, a comet whizzing by for an eve, in clouds which look like they belong on a gospel album cover.

In 2005, after Hurricane Wilma, south Florida had no power for days. In the *Palm Beach Post* newsroom, reporters were being dispatched to cover fuel shortages, the president's visit, hospitals running on generators.

I asked to write about the stars, which had lit up as cities fell to black. I was delighted when the editors agreed it was important to show readers a silver lining.

I wrote a story headlined, "Power of Universe: A Nightly Light Show," which began:

Light a candle rather than curse the darkness.

No. Leave the candle. Go out, look up, marvel in the darkness.

STARS!

I have a picture book of images taken by the Hubble Telescope. Images of infinity, beyond our dome of sky. Of things millions of light years away.

I remember clearly the images, but not what the images are, largely because it's incomprehensible to me.

Incomprehensible that the universe is so vast that all of Earth is a dot. A period at the end of a sentence, in a book a million pages long.

Whoa.

Whoa!

We almost didn't have those pictures. When the Hubble was launched into space, the first images beamed back to Earth were blurry. (Talk about an "ah shit" moment!)

The Hubble's lens had been ground incorrectly. By how much?

Two microns. One-fiftieth of the thickness of a piece of paper.

NASA dispatched an astronaut named Story (how lovely) to spacewalk out and fix it.

Later, another astronaut had to remove thirty-two tiny screws to replace a battery pack. While wearing what amounted to oven mitts. Even a slight nick in the spacesuit could kill him. He spoke of ignoring the earth below and the black vacuum in which he floated. He focused instead on one screw at a time.

One task.

One day.

What NASA does is awe-inspiring to me. I mean true jaw-dropping awe, and very few things in life move me like that.

How serendipitous, then, that July 8, 2011, less than three weeks after my diagnosis, was one of NASA's most storied events: the final space shuttle launch.

Most all my life I had lived in south Florida, a mere three-hour drive from the launch site in Cape Canaveral. At launch time, I had always dropped everything and dashed outside or to the window in my office in West Palm Beach, hoping to see the vessel—small as a star from that distance—blaze up the northern sky.

Yet I had never seen it up close.

Go, a voice inside my head told me. Don't feel sorry for yourself. Don't dwell on the muscle mass in your lower left arm. Fulfill a personal dream, by Jove, and see the shuttle *Atlantis* lift off.

I threw myself into the experience, reading everything I could find on the launch—the farewells, the reminiscences, the discoveries in its thirty years of flying, and the economic hardships caused by the end.

I read that a NASA executive hung a Dr. Seuss quote in his office to keep things in perspective: "Don't cry because it's over. Smile because it happened."

I will always remember that line.

The launch was not a sure thing. It had already been scrubbed once. As an astrophysicist on Space.com explained, the weather at four different sites around the world had to be "cross-correlated with myriad other factors, and extruded through a complex web of contingency requirements, boundary conditions, and constraints."

The weather forecast for July 8 was poor. Odds of a launch only 30 percent.

I set out anyway, for that is the way to experience: to go. With me was my seven-year-old son Wesley. My other children, Aubrey and Marina, were visiting John's parents in Pennsylvania.

Wesley and I drove the evening before to my friend Nancy's house in Orlando. Then, expecting full gridlock, we rose with Nancy and her children before dawn. We drove in a two-car caravan to the top of a parking garage in Cocoa Beach and found a bird's-eye view of the shuttle, if it launched, and the endless sky overhead.

We turned on NPR to listen to the play-by-play. It was cloudy, and a launch was far from guaranteed. We waited. Chatted. Enjoyed the uncertainty.

The poet Rainer Maria Rilke wrote: "Don't search for the answers, which could not be given to you now, because you would not be able to live them. And the point is to live everything. Live the questions now. Perhaps then, someday far in the future, you will gradually, without even noticing it, live your way into the answer."

I thought of my new uncertainty: How long can I live with ALS?

I thought: "Don't search for answers. Live the question."

Enjoy life more because of the uncertainty, not less.

Our parking lot was packed. We milled round and met people from all over the United States, some on bucket-list trips. Someone turned on music. A man came around selling cans of beer.

We went to the nearby surf shop to show the kids the huge saltwater tank with a shark inside. A friend of Nancy's had joined us with her two children. In the chaos of five kids, Wesley wandered off. It took us a few minutes to locate him—playing on the escalator. Completely enthralled by a moving staircase.

By midmorning, *Atlantis* was fueled and ready to go. We climbed atop my minivan, standing on its roof. Wesley was amazed. We were on top of the van!

"You'll dent the metal," someone yelled up to me.

"Who cares? It's history!" I replied.

We waited, listening to tributes and retrospectives. Will it launch? Won't it? The uncertainty was the joy.

The countdown began. T minus one minute.

The countdown stopped at thirty-one seconds to liftoff.

A few minutes later, without warning, the shuttle appeared in the clouds.

"I see it! I see it!" I yelled.

We stood on the dented roof and cheered.

We could not feel the shuttle rumble the ground. We could not see the orange explosion that launched it into space.

But we felt its wonder.

And smiled, though it was over.

Smiled because it happened.

Afterward we walked beside the ocean, abuzz with wonder, letting the traffic clear out. It didn't work. Even in the evening, the roads were packed. I drove at five miles an hour, thinking about the shuttle. Of NASA's central message, the one a part of its very existence: Reach out. Explore. Dream big. Go.

Go now.

The big questions rose before me: Where do I want to go? How do I want to live? What is the central message of my life?

The small questions too: Where are my photographs? What will I eat when my tongue fails? And what about this maxed-out bladder?

Ugh. I had to pee.

There was no chance to pull over in the traffic jam. Besides, with my weak arms and fingers, public restrooms weren't as easy as they used to be.

You have the bladder of a camel, I thought. You'll make it back to Nancy's.

I did. I held my bladder for three hours, all the way to Nancy's house.

She wasn't there. Wesley and I had left her car behind us on the road somewhere.

I tried the doors. Locked.

I looked around, thought about waiting . . . then shrugged.

Half an hour later, when Nancy and her family arrived, Wesley and I were bobbing in the pool, fully dressed, huge smiles on our faces.

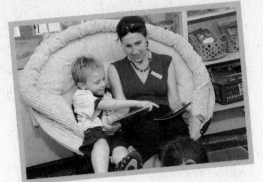

Wesley

After that trip, it would take me a while to retrain Wesley that we don't usually swim in clothes. Not near as long, though, as it took us to get him to wear a swimsuit in the first place.

Which I suppose I should explain.

Wesley was my third child. I was thirty-six when I had him, and I knew he was my last. Yet when the doctor offered to tie my tubes during the C-section delivery, I declined, not wanting that period of my life to be over.

I appreciated his infancy, even the sleepless nights, as only an experienced mother can. Wesley was clingy, which I loved. If he fell asleep on my breast, I'd stare at him for an hour. *Remember this!* I told myself over and over.

He didn't crawl much, unlike Marina and Aubrey, but he started talking early. By the time he turned one, Wesley was saying whole sentences, like "Let's go see the hippopotamus today."

"He's a genius!" John said.

As we realized later, he was imitating sounds. He had no idea what he was saying, or even that he was using words.

His behavioral issues started at three. He slammed doors over and over. Flipped light switches on and off compulsively. Ignored everything John and I said. I used to bang a pot behind his head to see if he could hear, he was so oblivious to our voices. He always jumped.

The situation reached a head that Christmas, when we took the kids to a fancy mall to see Santa. There were Christmas lights, Christmas trees, giant snowflakes glittering on strings, hundreds of kids and shoppers, at least two competing sets of Christmas carols . . . and Wesley fritzed out.

We were waiting in the long, long Santa line, and he could not stand still or stop screaming. John and I walked him around and took him into stores. No good. Wesley tried to climb into the fountain.

We gave up and dragged the kids to our minivan, all three now complaining. I was a smoker, but I only smoked a few cigarettes a day and rarely in front of the children. After an hour of Wesley's behavior, though, I was at my wits' end.

"Mom, what are you doing?" yelled eight-year-old Marina when she looked out of the van and saw me smoking.

"Mom!! You can't litter!" Marina hollered.

I picked up the butt and threw it on the van floor. Wesley was screaming and struggling so much, I sat on the floor at his feet to comfort him.

We were halfway to the next, more subdued mall when we smelled smoke. The cigarette butt was smoldering on the carpet of John's company car.

We screeched into the Palm Beach Mall: me beating out

the smoking carpet; John furious and cursing; Marina whining and snapping at a forlorn Aubrey, "There's no Santa, stupid"; Wesley berserk.

We trundled the kids across the semi-deserted mall to Santa's "Wonderland." No line, but Santa was going on break. The elf tried to stop us, but Santa looked over at our family and said, "No, no. I'll take this one."

John and I pushed Aubrey up with one hand, trying to control Wesley with our others. Aubrey was five, a little shy, with a lisp. He stopped short, turned to John with a confused look, and said, "Daddy, why is Santa bwown?"

That bwown Santa smiled. He had more Christmas spirit than all of us put together.

After the holidays (a series of disasters), I insisted on taking Wesley for an evaluation. I remember the psychologist saying, "He looks at you. That's good," and me thinking, Oh shit!

The psychologist called us back to her office a week later. There was one soft light and a box of Kleenex by the sofa. "I believe Wesley has Asperger's," she said.

Again, I was clueless. "What's Asperger's?"

"It's a form of autism."

I reached for the Kleenex, already crying. That was and shall remain the worst day of my life. I still can't drive past the building where Wesley was diagnosed.

Two years later, Wesley had made tremendous progress. It took a lot of paperwork and planning, a lot of long nights and phone calls, but I had fast-tracked Wesley into the local pre-K program for children with special needs at Meadow Park Elementary. The staff worked miracles, tamping down Wesley's odd behaviors, focusing him to learn.

He entered the regular kindergarten there in 2009. The orientation was held in the library, about a month after I noticed my withered hand—and a week after I first heard those three letters: ALS.

As the teachers talked, most of the kids colored quietly beside their parents. One child even appeared to be taking notes. Wesley scampered around the library, pulling books off the shelves and egging on another little boy to chase him.

My leg muscle started quivering. My ankle was propped on my knee, and I saw my calf twitch, a primary symptom of ALS. *New York Times* writer Dudley Clendinen, who died of ALS, described these twitches in the most beautiful way, "like butterflies fluttering underneath the skin."

I clenched the muscles to stop the shaking. But when I unclenched, the butterflies returned.

"Mom," Wesley called in his loudest voice. He always used his loudest voice. "Mom! Mom!"

I smiled. Sure, Wesley was pulling books off shelves at kindergarten orientation. But he was also asking another child to play. Yes, in the wrong setting, at the wrong time, and way too loud, but Wesley was asking. I felt so happy for Wesley in that moment, so optimistic, that nothing in the world could bring me down, including a twitchy calf.

"It's Google twitches," John said that night. "You read about ALS symptoms on the Internet, and now you are experiencing them."

It's going to be all right, I told myself. Wesley is going to be all right.

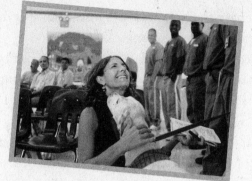

Animals and Expectations

In August 2010, we adopted a dog. In many ways, it was a responsibility I didn't need. My muscle problems were spreading, and I was still working full-time while raising three energetic kids.

But Marina and Aubrey kvetched constantly about not having a dog. Not having a dog and not having cable, in that order. The horror!

"It's just not normal, Mom," Marina complained.

"I have a fish, Mom," Aubrey said with a sigh. "That is not a real pet."

And Wesley, poor Wesley. His behavior had improved, but the little guy remained distant and disconnected. He talked nonstop, but never a conversation. He could watch over and over his beloved *Backyardigans* episodes, but he rarely expressed emotion, love, or affection for anything aside from his little stuffed Piglet.

Hugging him was much like hugging a tree.

"You have to find a way into his world," the doctor had said when she diagnosed him.

We live close to a small zoo. For years, it had been Wesley's favorite outing. The animals didn't require him to look them in the eye or order him around. He drew humans as stick figures with bubble heads, but even at six years old he drew extraordinary pictures of dolphins and dogs and bears. Animals, I knew, made Wesley comfortable.

The dog, I told myself, was a gift for him.

I didn't admit how much I needed the distraction. Or how much I craved the attention of an animal. I just thought: the more affection around the children, especially Wesley, the better.

Enter man's best friend!

It had been a decade since I had a dog, a fifty-pound Rottweiler mutt, Alva, a stray my friend Nancy and I took in during grad school. Alva had a host of quirks from street life. She ate everything, including garbage, shoes, and felt-tip markers—and routinely excreted a steamy pile upon the one square yard of carpet in our house.

She got cancer and had to have her leg amputated. You have never seen a happier three-legged dog than Alva.

But in my condition, rolling the dice on a street mutt like Alva was not an option. And puppies, they are like babies, right? I wasn't doing that again.

Thus began the search for a dog that needed a home, but already knew how to behave in one. A real pet for Marina and Aubrey. A friend for Wesley.

A comfort for a mother in need.

So where did I find the right dog? The one to warm my little boy's life?

The coldest place of all: prison.

One morning, I was looking up a murderer on the Florida Department of Corrections website. Yes, I did that often. Part of my job as a reporter. Past the "Most Wanted" notices, blotter descriptions, and pictures of officers in riot gear was a ticker: "Will you adopt me?" and photos of dogs graduating from training programs in Florida's prisons.

The dogs, rescued from area shelters, lived with inmate trainers for eight weeks. They were taught to stay, lie down, release, walk on a leash, not enter or exit a doorway without hearing the command to do so. They were crate-trained, potty-trained, and vaccinated.

They were . . . perfect!

Within five minutes, I was on the phone with Sandy Christy, director of DAWGS (Developing Adoptable Dogs With Good Sociability) in Prison.

Ms. Christy recommended a dog in training. Gracie was sixty pounds, but docile, obedient, and easy to command. "She is the star of the class," Ms. Christy said.

She sent pictures—Gracie sitting, lying, standing, tongue wagging. She was muscular and white, with a pink nose and gold eyes. She certainly looked like a lovebug.

But Gracie was five hundred miles away, in a prison near the Florida Panhandle town of White City.

I looked at the photos of Gracie. Imagined the kids flocking to be near her. Imagined her chewing my Ferragamo heels. Imagined her swimming in the pool, then plopping down on my Ethan Allen sofa. Imagined her lying beside the children at night, snacking on their duvets. I imagined Gracie following little Wesley around when he retreated from the rest of us.

I talked to my father. He already fielded daily pickup, drop-off, babysitting, and home-improvement requests. Would he take on, when necessary, the responsibility of a dog?

"I think it's a great idea," Dad said. "I'll go with you to pick her up."

John was the wild card, one day strident about not getting a dog— "It's too much, Susan" —the next gushing about the cutest little bulldog he saw at a shelter.

"Are we crazy?" I asked John. "To adopt, sight unseen, a dog five hundred miles away?"

"Remember," he said, "someone adopted you sight unseen."

A one-thousand-mile round trip later to prison and back, Marina and Aubrey charged out our front door.

"Gracie! Gracie!" they squealed.

Wesley hung back, not wanting to come out of the house. But once the dog was inside, he joined the squealing pet-fest. Gracie, poor thing, urinated on the carpet.

No bother.

Now, Wesley will never spontaneously hug a human being. Never. But that night, Wesley climbed right inside the kennel with Gracie, sat beside her, patted her (at times bordering on pounding her), talking to her IN A VOICE LIKE THIS.

And *thump, thump, thump* went Gracie's tail.

"Look, Mom, she has sharp teeth!" Wesley said, peeling back her top and bottom lips. Gracie gave him a big lick on the cheek.

"Can I sleep with Gracie?" Wesley asked.

And just like that, Gracie was part of the family. The one

who chased lizards. The expert digger (we joke the prisoners must have taught her that one). The one my kids greeted first in the morning and kissed last at night.

Within days, Wesley and Gracie were constant companions. When Gracie rolled on her back, inviting a belly scratch, Wesley obliged.

He no longer washed his hands after his French toast sticks, wanting Gracie to lick the syrup off instead.

He read her picture books, helped dress her in her Halloween costume (a duck), and wanted her in the bathroom when he took a bath.

Wesley loved to let her lick his face, relishing the ones right smack-dab on the mouth.

"Yuck." I sighed.

But wonderful, for Wesley had never relished physical contact before.

I used to sing the children to sleep every night. I would sing soft and low, almost in a hum, until Wesley settled down.

John nearly cries when he thinks of it now. He told me he stood outside Wesley's door for years, listening to me sing. That's one of the rare requests John has made of me: to record my voice singing that song, before it slipped away.

Gracie became my surrogate song.

"Go lie down, Wesley," I would say to him. "Be still and silent."

"Then Gracie will come?"

"Yes."

He would zip into his bed, pull his Thomas the Train blanket over him, eyes wide open in the nightlight, waiting.

I would walk Gracie in, until I could no longer walk. I

would watch as she hopped on Wesley's bed, took one last lick at his face, then curled up beside him, closer than I ever could, and fell asleep.

Wesley's eighth birthday was September 9, 2011. It was the first major life event after my ALS diagnosis in June, and I wanted a quiet time. So did he. Wesley is most comfortable alone with Gracie. A swarm of party guests and noise would be unpleasant.

I knew the perfect plan: John, Wesley, and I would spend his birthday at the best zoo in the area, Metro Zoo, an hour and a half away in Miami, Florida.

"There are elephants at the big zoo," I told Wesley. "Wanna go see them in Miami?"

"Yes! I want to go to Your-ami!" he said.

I laid down the rules ahead of time with John. "We see the animals Wesley wants to see. Let him lead us to kingdom come."

Metro Zoo has these wonderful four-wheeled cart bicycles with a lemon-yellow canopy to shield the sun. We rented one, and John pedaled us to the Asian elephants.

Then across the zoo to the African elephants.

Then back again to the Asian ones to look at their ears. And back to the African ones to note the difference.

And back and forth again to note their heads.

And once again to compare their size.

We pedaled around all day, sipping lemonade, eating cotton candy, looking at elephants. Wesley was in heaven.

And so was I.

I didn't have a plan for my year, beyond living with joy. I

just grasped the opportunities that arose: the wonder of the space shuttle. The simplicity of a day at the zoo. The peace of lying down with Gracie.

Those experiences were precious, I realized, because of Wesley. He helped me appreciate Gracie, even when she dug up our backyard. He taught me that African elephants have Africa-shaped ears.

Because of him, I know those yellow four-person bicycles are made in Italy and too expensive for a middle-class family to afford (believe me, I tried).

If not for Wesley, I wouldn't have appreciated how exciting it was, on the day the space shuttle launched, to stand on top of our van.

Those memories remain crystal sharp for me. Every time I think of them, I smile. When I am paralyzed, they will be my comfort and strength.

But what would Wesley remember? That was the question.

When you are facing death, you long to leave something behind. I wanted to plant memories, but what Wesley remembered was entirely random, one of his Aspie quirks. Often, he didn't seem to remember at all.

In late August 2012, more than a year after the trip, I began writing about our adventure to see the space shuttle—the dented roof, the uncertainty, the wonder when it soared.

Curious, I asked Wesley, in a nonleading way, if he remembered our adventure.

He twirled his long, blond hair in his fingers. "Yup," he said, popping the last sound like he always does. "Yeh-puh. I remember."

I asked: "Who was there?"

He rattled off the names of Nancy's family. I thought he might be naming people by rote, as he often does. Then he added two names—Samantha and Brooke—Nancy's friend's children. The only time we met them was that day.

"Where did we watch?" I asked.

"On top of the van."

Wesley smiled. As did I, with delight.

A few weeks later, he drew a gorgeous picture of Cindy the dolphin in black magic marker. It is framed now, and hangs over our dining table.

Mission accomplished, I think when I see it.

Wesley's garden is already growing.

The Yukon

October

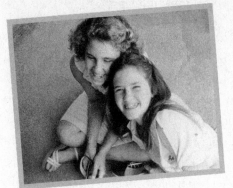

Auroras

I f you were dying, what would you do? What would you see? Who would you spend your last year with?

I knew I wanted to travel. Travel had always been magic to me, the essence of life. So many happy times were defined by where I'd been.

Since my children were born, I had put off special trips, always thinking, I'm too busy now, but when the children are older, when the job slows down . . .

Now the excuses were gone. There would be no more waiting. The world was open to me, and I could go anywhere.

An-y-where.

But where? What had I never seen that had, even from a distance, filled me with awe? The Great Wall of China? The Taj Mahal of India?

Or the Atacama Desert of Chile? They say the Atacama is like being on the surface of the moon. Astronomers have found asteroid particles there that contain the same amino acids humans have. Oh! The mental magic the Atacama would be.

Or should I go on the most romantic getaway I could imagine: in Spain, at a monastery turned luxury hotel on a cliff overlooking the sea? A place to make love while still able, to experience those earnest, luscious tremblings on velvet.

It was my best friend, Nancy Maass Kinnally, who focused my attention. Ever since our trip to New Orleans, when I acknowledged my condition for the first time, she had been trying to plan something exotic for the two of us: the trip of a lifetime.

Nancy and I were born two weeks apart and raised three miles apart. We met as eleven-year-olds at Palm Beach Public Junior High School and have been best friends since. We went to college at the University of North Carolina together and to graduate school at the University of Florida.

Nancy was always Ms. Phi Beta Kappa. And I was Ms. I Tappa Kegga.

We balanced one another. We clicked largely because we laughed at the exact same things and could shut each other up when need be.

We shared a love of adventure and had traveled abroad, including Hungary and Peru. We visited Macchu Picchu on the summer solstice in 1997 and were surrounded by California New Agers. (It's, like, the sol-stice, man.) The Californians kept whining that the food was not organic.

So we escaped and climbed the opposite peak, Huayna Picchu, for peace and quiet and a view of the ancient home of Incan emperors.

I was five months pregnant. I slipped and nearly fell.

Yet we laughed the whole time, and haven't stopped laughing since.

Today—thirty-four years, five kids, and umpteen personal crises later—Nancy and I are still those silly seventh-graders, chuckling about boys and bodily functions, crackin' jokes.

It was going to be pretty hard to top the experiences we had already had together. But Nancy was adamant it was going to happen.

She contacted her brother, who offered his luxury apartment in Buenos Aires. A European city in South America, in a lavish pied-a-terre. A base to explore South America.

No, Buenos Aires was lovely, no doubt, but I had no connection there.

A friend in Goa, India, invited us to visit. Another friend from junior high school had moved to India and been ordained a Buddhist nun. Perhaps a visit to her monastery at the same time? And learn to meditate?

Nancy really wanted India.

"Seriously?" I said. "Can you see me in a Buddhist monastery? 'I can't meditate now—it's cocktail hour!' "

The inspiration came to me on an afternoon in late September. It was breezy, but still Florida: hot as blazes. Nancy and I were standing on a floating dock in West Palm Beach, awaiting friends in a boat.

I was already having trouble walking on terra firma. The slightly swaying dock was a reminder of my future, when even standing would be hard. I focused on the sky—balance, Susan, balance—and thought of auroras.

One of nature's most spectacular phenomena, seen near

the poles of the earth, a sky light show often green and white, at times red, pink, purple, and blue.

The rainbow of the night sky.

I was transfixed the first time I read of auroras in Admiral Richard Byrd's book *Alone*, his account of the months he spent in Antarctic darkness, his neglected senses expanding to exquisite sensitivity.

Byrd wrote of a giant elliptical green aurora he witnessed:

> Scintillating in the sky was what appeared to be a drapery hanging over the South Pole composed of brilliant light rays . . .
>
> Overhead the aurora began to change shape and became a great lustrous serpent and the folds in the curtain over the pole began to undulate as if stirred by a celestial presence. Star after star disappeared as the serpentine folds covered them.
>
> I was left with the tingling feeling that I had witnessed a scene denied to other mortal men.

I am a spiritual person. I believe in God. I believe in forces beyond us in the universe, wonders we are too small to comprehend.

In phenomena like the auroras, we glimpse these wonders. For a moment in their presence, we can sense, and feel, and see.

"The Yukon Territory? In winter?" Nancy gaped when I told her my wish. I had never spoken of this fascination before. And Nancy hates the cold.

"What happened to India? Why can't India be on your bucket list?" (She was half kidding. Maybe.)

"Of course," she said, "I will do whatever you wish."

Just then our friends Lisa and Anatole picked us up in their boat—a little teak-adorned one formerly owned by Jimmy Buffett.

We spent the day enjoying the best of Florida: sunning, swimming, joining a gaggle of other boats at a nearby island where people crank stereos, pop beer cans, and display their thongs and tattoos.

Lisa is a judge, weighing grave matters all week long. It was a delight to see her kick back and relax as we watched the skin pageant before us.

We were enjoying it so, in fact, that we failed to notice a massive thunderstorm until it was upon us. My friends scrambled to get our gear to shore, where we could wait out the storm. Unable to help, I sat on the boat near its metal canopy. I felt the electricity in the air, and thought how perfect it would be if lightning struck me.

I asked to remain on the boat.

Nancy and Lisa wouldn't hear of it. They helped me to shore. Together with a too-friendly man we had just met, we huddled on the beach, arms around one another, as cold rain beat down and lightning struck nearby.

I have no idea the odds of being struck by lightning.

Or the odds that I would be struck with ALS.

It doesn't matter. It can happen to anyone. Lightning strikes in the middle of paradise. ALS cuts down a famous baseball player, an older man, a son, a daughter, a mother in the prime of life.

I had accepted. I would move on.

To the Yukon Territory. To auroras.

Off the boat, and into the arms of my friends.

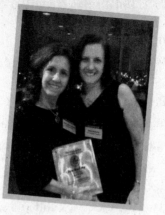

Thank You

There was one thing I needed to do before the Yukon. A heartbreaking thing: quit the journalism job I loved.

For more than a year, I had been struggling, improvising solutions for my failing health.

When I could no longer lift my laptop, I asked other people to get it out of my bag, place it on my lap, and open it for me.

When my precise keyboard choreography went kerflooey, and my pinkie finger would no longer reach the *p*—I began to hunt-and-peck.

And I began to miss deadlines. I shall rephrase to say, I began to miss more deadlines.

It unsettled me. I banged out updates as best I could with about six working fingers, even tweeting from the courtroom. The *Palm Beach Post* was counting on me. We were in a recession, especially in the newspaper biz, and I was taking up a slot that could have gone to someone with two hands.

I began to lie awake at night, worried I wasn't pulling my weight. That I wasn't a top-notch reporter any more. Slowly, I began to dread going to the job I adored.

But how could I quit? Being a journalist was my identity. To lose it would be to lose a piece of myself.

And what about money? I had big plans, but I wasn't sure I could afford them. In fact, I wasn't sure we could pay our monthly expenses without my job.

Nancy, as always, stepped in. I want you to understand this, because it's important. Every day, when I need something, John is there. Every moment I despair, the thought of my children comforts me. And at every turning point in my life, when someone has stepped forward, it has been Nancy.

Nancy worked in communications for the Florida Bar Foundation in Orlando. After my diagnosis with ALS, she figured there must be legal provisions to help a sick person like me, and she suggested a few local lawyers who could look into the matter.

The Legal Aid lawyers, John and Stephanie, explained to me the Americans with Disabilities Act. They told me about medical leave of absence.

John went through all my paperwork, all that HR stuff from the office you stick in a drawer and never look at twice, and found something: I had a life insurance policy through the *Post*. A pretty big one. If I was terminally ill—yes to that one, unfortunately—I could take 70 percent of my benefits early. Not just early, but immediately. Yukon, here I come!

The process took almost three months—all through the summer, as I watched the space shuttle with Wesley and embraced my future and planned our birthday trip to the zoo.

The whole time, I said next to nothing to my colleagues. I just kept working.

I worked harder than ever, in fact, determined to do the job the same way I always had.

And for a while I did. I worked so effectively, and with such joy, I began to wonder: Maybe I can continue?

Then I fell down the stairs.

I had been pushing myself, refusing to give in to weakness. But I pushed too far and, on the stairs outside the public prosecutors' offices, my leg gave out.

I crashed down. Didn't have the arm strength to stop my fall and tumbled to the bottom.

By the time I was helped to my feet, there was blood running down my left leg. "You need a doctor," someone said.

"No," I replied. "I'm late for an interview."

The interview was with the top prosecutor. He was no fan of my reporting. When I walked in, he gave me the usual cold look. That I'll-talk-to-you-cuz-I-gotta-but-I'm-not-going-to-like-it stare.

Then he saw my leg.

"Are you hurt? You're hurt. Let's do this later."

I realized right then: there was no doing something later. I would never again be stronger than I was today.

"No," I said, "Let's do it now."

Not long after, my editor phoned me. "What the hell is wrong with you?" she said.

"Call my lawyer," I told her.

I didn't mean to be rude. The words had come to my mind—*I have ALS*—but I couldn't say them. Not without breaking down in tears, and that was something I couldn't do.

A few days later, I was on a cigarette break with Judge Barry Cohen, a man I had written about for years. We often lunched together in the courthouse cafeteria, along with other judges and attorneys I admired.

I don't know why I said it. I didn't plan it at all. Suddenly, I turned to him and said, "I don't think I'm coming back."

Then I turned and walked away, as fast as I could with my dignity intact.

That time, I did cry. Because I loved that job, and I had just admitted to myself that it was gone.

I took a medical leave of absence in mid-August. Two weeks later, I won an award from the Florida Bar for my tweeting and web updates. It was statewide recognition, one of the highest accomplishments for a court journalist like me.

The award was given at a major dinner, attended by journalists, attorneys, and members of the Florida Supreme Court. My boss at the *Palm Beach Post*, Nick Moschella, wanted me to go. He thought it would be good for the newspaper, and for me.

But the event was in Tallahassee, the state capital, five hundred miles away on the other end of the state. No way could I drive in my condition, and the trip was last-minute because nobody had been checking my work mailbox. The plane ticket cost $700.

I couldn't justify the expense; not when I knew I wasn't coming back.

"Please use the money to send a reporter on assignment," I told Nick. "I'll pay my own way to Tallahassee."

I decided to take the bus.

I had ridden buses often in other countries. But I had never been on a Greyhound bus in America. Go for it, Susan, I told myself. Have an adventure.

The trip was long, boring, and miserable. I think it took eight hours. For half of that time, I sat across from a heavy metal band. They spent their time complaining to their manager, loudly, on a cell phone, about having to take the stinking bus.

They meant the stinking part literally.

At one stop, I fell over backward as I struggled on the bus's stairs. "Man, she is wasted," I heard the heavy metal dudes say.

I arrived on the day of the awards presentation. Bedraggled. Besotted. The bus! In my condition. What was I thinking?

Nancy let me crash in her hotel room. A bath, a nap, and a friend: that picked up my spirits. That afternoon, amid cries of "Let's go for it," we Googled our way into a Yukon vacation and booked the tickets.

Aurora borealis, here we come!

That evening, I glammed up in a nice dress. Put on my makeup and favorite necklace, made from a medal of Saint Andreas. And, unfortunately, my flats. Just before taking medical leave from work, I had fallen coming out of my house and broken my clavicle. That was when I realized my legs were too weak for high heels.

The ceremony was on the top floor of the capitol building, in a room with window walls and a 360-degree view. At sunset, my favorite time of day. All the big wheels in my business were there, including a few justices on the State Supreme Court.

The moment didn't strike me, though, until a friend, Neil Skene, told the story of my last year, right up to and including the bus trip. As I walked up to get my award, the applause started. When I turned to face the crowd, I realized they were all standing.

I knew it wasn't for my tweets. It was for twenty years.

It moved me.

I can't remember my acceptance speech, but I think it was this: "Thank you."

The next morning, I took the bus back home. A month later, I was on my way to the Yukon with Nancy.

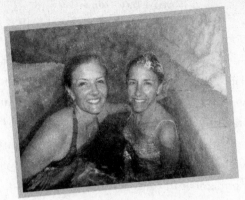

The Northern Lights

We had selected a site five hours below the Arctic Circle in Canada's Yukon Territory: a town called Whitehorse and an outfit, Northern Tales Travel Service, which specialized in taking aurora seekers on their quest.

No inside information, just a Google search. Their website's photos of a glorious aurora and a warm cabin intrigued me.

It certainly looked like a place for a "scene denied to other mortal men," as Byrd wrote. "A place where neglected senses turned to exquisite sensitivity."

Nancy and I made a grand trip of it. Flying first to San Francisco then Vancouver, leaving warmer-weather clothes at the hotel for our return. Whitehorse was a two-and-a-half-hour flight from Vancouver, mostly north.

We cracked up at the tropical silk flower arrangements at the Air North ticket counter. I asked the agent about the weather up in Whitehorse: "Twenty below and snowing," he said.

The cold literally took my breath away. When I stepped outside in Whitehorse, my air refused to come out. I wondered if nostrils could freeze shut.

At least we had Northern Tales agent Stefan Wackerhagen to heat us up. Stefan was a German dogsledder and outdoorsman who looked like a rugged Anderson Cooper. "Yay!" Nancy and I telegraphed to each other.

He took us to our hotel, the Best Western Gold Rush Inn, then handed us two large red duffels full of the winter-weather gear we had rented. We went to our rooms and suited up for the first of three nights of aurora viewing.

Or, rather, Nancy did. With my weak hands, I hadn't a prayer of zipping, tugging, lacing, or buttoning anything. After she finished with her own tugging and zipping, Nancy tugged me into my skintight running pants, my jeans, my wool socks, goose-down bib overalls, a nylon skintight undershirt, a cotton turtleneck, a cashmere sweater, a down parka, and a pair of heavy lace-up winter boots.

"What's the number-one pickup line in the Yukon?" I asked. " 'I'm sure you're not nearly as fat as you look in that parka.' "

Over and over on the trip, Nancy would suit and unsuit me, at one point declaring the nylon undershirt "toxic waste."

I blamed it on the cheap deodorant she kept putting on me.

About ten in the evening, our guide drove us a half hour outside Whitehorse along the Alaskan Highway. We sped into pitch-black, the powdery snow skittering across the road in the headlights. Turned off onto an unmarked snow-packed path through the trees and parked beside a small cabin in the middle of nowhere.

To the north was an open white field, with benches at the side.

And above a vast expanse of sky for Mother Nature to paint on.

That first night the winds whooshed so much we could not build a fire, and we passed the hours inside the cabin, around a black wood-burning stove, glowing orange.

Tacked up on a cabin wall were pelts of fox and bear, the bear shot on the property (a fun fact I really didn't need to hear).

On another wall was a world map where light seekers pinned their hometowns, some as far away as Tahiti, South Africa, and New Zealand. A wooden bench with pillows ringed the cabin. There was a snack bar with ten different kinds of hot tea, coffee and hot chocolate, cookies, chips, and marshmallows.

But no northern lights. That vast expanse of sky remained choked in clouds.

Now what does one do in the Yukon winter when not standing in a field in the middle of the night?

Northern Tales offered day trips—wildlife preserve, dog-sledding tours, or a visit to a hot spring. So the next day, Nancy put an extra layer on me: a swimsuit.

Takhini Hot Springs is an outdoor oasis fed by water percolating deep in the earth, then returning to the surface laden with minerals and 104 degrees.

Nancy and I were the only visitors there that afternoon. I stared at the steps leading into the pool. The handrail was on the left side, my weaker side.

Suddenly, this struck me as a bad idea. In warm weather maybe, but not lumbering in a wet swimsuit at ten below. I envisioned Nancy in a permafrosted bikini struggling to hoist me up from the frozen floor.

"I'm not going in."

"What? Susan! Come on!"

Back and forth like that a few times, then Nancy went off to ask for help from the gorgeous man at the front desk. I overheard him telling her about the eighty-year-old arthritic lady he helps out of the pools. I envisioned him hoisting my failing self.

No way, I thought.

Then I heard Nancy say to him something that moved me: "I've never seen her like that before."

"Okay, okay, I'll do it," I hollered from the changing room.

For the umpteenth time, Nancy undressed me—parka, overalls, three shirts, two pants. We headed down the cold-creaking walkway in our swimsuits, laying our towels on a frost-covered rack.

Nancy stepped down the stairs into the water. "Ooh, kinda feels like it's burning you!" she said.

She turned around to help me. We glided in silently with hardly a ripple.

I gasped and clenched my teeth until I realized the water was not singeing me. It was perfectly hot, steaming in the freezing air. We found the spouts where the hot spring water flows into the pool and sat on a bench beside them, up to our necks in a thermal winter wonderland.

The hot springs were a semicircle, offering a fish-eye view of the surroundings. A forest of frosted fir trees. A motionless sky of clouds. It was so quiet, you could hear branches groaning under the weight of the snow.

One by one, the droplets of water in our hair froze. Slowly, Nancy's hair turned white, until she looked like a little old lady.

I thought of sitting beside her at the hospital one distant day awaiting the birth of her first grandchild. Of being beside her at the graduations and weddings and funerals to come.

I had been consumed since my diagnosis with preparing for death: making voice recordings for my children, planning trips, obsessing over finances, trying to preserve my family's ability to live with joy without me. But in those moments, I saw the future on the face of my friend—and me a part of it.

The clouds opened, an azure sky aglow in the sunset, and inside me returned a sense of hope.

The second night of aurora viewing was clear as glass and still. Our guide was a Cuban gentleman, Leandro Font. A part-time guide, a new one, who himself had not seen the lights out at the cabin site.

So there we were, two Floridians and a Cuban, waiting. Staring into the darkness, trying to divine the miracle of the sub-Arctic.

We saw a light at the horizon, moving behind a stand of trees. We trained our cosmic zoom and held our breaths. It was a car.

"I tink dat's de northern headlights," Font said.

After a few hours, I went inside the cabin and lay down by the glowing stove. I awoke from a dead sleep to Font hollering: "It's coming! It's coming!"

I wobbled out to the field, Nancy yelling: "Look! Look! See it there!"

There it was—a horizontal band about 30 degrees high in the night sky. A ghost of the heavens. Is it green or white? I was wondering, when I tripped and fell over in the snow, whacking my head on the way down.

By the time Nancy and Leandro hoisted me up, the light was gone.

On our final day in Whitehorse, Stefan took us dogsledding at Muktuk Kennels, home to 120 or so Alaskan huskies. We were ensconced in our winter space suits and boots when Stefan said, "I don't think those boots will be warm enough. We'll get you some bunny boots instead."

Bunny boots are a lace-up white rubber creation of the U.S. military for minus-forty-degree weather. They are like strapping two bricks to each foot and about as comfortable.

"Do you have any physical problems?" our amiable Muktuk guide Tori asked Nancy as we suited up.

"Oh, yeah," said Nancy. "Exercise-induced asthma in cold weather."

We laughed and stepped out of the tackhouse into minus 10 degrees. Tori and Nancy harnessed eight dogs and swaddled me in the sled—a cushion at my back, a hot water bottle at my torso, and a sleeping bag over me. They zipped up the canvas cover and pulled my wool turtleneck over my mouth and nose, leaving just my eyes peering out.

Tori gave Nancy a primer on operating a dogsled, a gaggle of unintelligible-to-me directions about brakes and snow hooks and vocal commands that only make sense to dogs. All I understood was: "Whatever you do, don't let go."

Last thing Tori said to Nancy: "There's a hill where you'll have to get off and run. The dogs can't pull all the weight."

"Wait . . . what?!?"

Too late. We were off.

We soon reached said hill. "Oh, God, I should have eaten my Wheaties," Nancy groaned.

She moved to the side of the sled and jogged up the snowy hill in her brick bunny boots. Her breathing became louder and shorter.

About halfway up I heard: "I wonder how far." Gasp. "We are." Gasp. "From." Gasp. "A hospital."

Nancy never let the sled go. She kept hold as it threatened to drag her along. She sounded on the edge of an asthma attack. Finally, at the top of the hill, she was able to catch her breath.

"You're buying me effing dinner," Nancy eked out.

We laughed and laughed the rest of the ride on level trail, the dogs pulling us through the white fir forest—pines and spruce rising around us in silence. The only sound the *pat, pat, pat* of thirty-two paws on the snow.

I had come to see the silent wonder of the sky. And found wonder in the silence right around me.

This is a dream, I thought. This is a dream.

Our final night of aurora viewing was a Friday, and we were joined by a dozen folks who came for the weekend. A Chinese family. A Japanese fashion designer inspired by Jack London novels. A couple from Toronto who said seeing the lights was a bucket-list trip.

I didn't ask them why, nor did I tell anyone my reasons.

I passed about my bottle of Hennessy, drank oodles of hot chocolate and hot tea. Stefan practiced taking souvenir pictures—long exposures where we would stand completely still while the camera captured the undulating curtain of lights behind us.

If only the lights would come.

I had stopped checking the auroral forecast the day before. I knew I couldn't change it. Why worry? What's meant to be was meant to be.

That's how my psychologist advised me to answer my children's questions. When they ask, "Mommy, are you going to die?" I answer: "I don't know what's meant to be."

But of course I hoped the lights would come.

I looked about the cabin at the framed photos of glorious green auroras. I thought of the delight and extraordinary kindness of every Canadian we met. I watched my dear friend giddily chatting up the ripped Anderson Cooper look-alike.

My friend who spent thousands of dollars to travel eight thousand miles to a freezing place she had zip-zero interest in going with zip-zero guarantee of seeing any stinkin' lights.

We waited until 3:00 a.m.

But it wasn't meant to be.

"Would you rather have seen the lights and not met all these people and not experienced all these things?" Nancy asked.

"No," I answered.

And then she reminded me: "It's the journey, not the destination, true?"

"True." I said. "A bit hackneyed, but true indeed."

She sighed. I smiled.

"Good night, my beautiful friend."

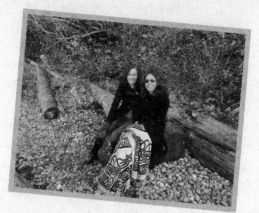

Wreck Beach

In the Yukon, the cold sapped me of energy. I noticed my feet dragging in the heavy boots and being exhausted after shivering. I hoped it was just that—the extreme cold.

In Vancouver, on the way home, I discovered otherwise. Back in the relative warmth, with fewer clothes and cute flats instead of boots, I still felt weak.

We had a one-day layover—hello Four Seasons!—so my friend Nick and his girlfriend Junmin took Nancy and me out for an afternoon. Nick was the producer of a television show on true crime. He had recently filmed a special on my favorite victim—gunshot survivor Heather Grossman, an inspiring quadriplegic I had written many newspaper articles about— and despite my slurred speech, he insisted I be involved.

Nick suggested a spot on the beach, with a view of Vancouver's bay and the surrounding hills. It was a sunny day, but chilly. We could build a fire, Nick said, and watch the sun set.

Perfect!

The entrance to Wreck Beach was a steep bank of stairs descending into forest. Fifty feet below, the stairs twisted out of sight. I could not see their end.

We started down. By the first landing, a canopy of cedar and fir trees covered the sky, with ferns and bushes—electric green—surrounding their trunks. There was a little snow on the steps. Leaves falling silently in the lush air. Spots of sunlight here and there.

A perfect place to fall in love, I thought.

We started down again, slowly, the stairs carpeted in autumn's slippery gift of gold and crimson.

We turned a bend, passed huckleberry and maples, more slippery stairs. The climate changed as we descended, along with the plants too. More ferns. More moisture. No snow.

I thought of how my physical therapist taught me to put my weaker left leg first, then follow with my right.

I parsed each step. Planting left, then right. One foot, then the other. Waiting for Nancy to join me on each step, so I could grab her if I slipped.

I tired. I sat on a bench with her, resting.

"Wanna turn back?" she asked.

"No."

Hundreds more steps, but I parsed them all, one foot after the other.

We arrived at the shore.

The spot was as divine as Nick described: the bay, the hills, and all Vancouver before us.

Nick lit a fire.

I was exhausted. Too tired to totter across the beach shoreline of polished stones. I sat on a driftwood log. It was cold in the wind. I wondered if we might have to call the fire department to haul me back up the steps. Nancy wondered too.

She covered my legs with a blanket. Eventually, they helped me to the fire.

Nick and Junmin talked of how they met. She had been a florist Nick often visited.

Telling, isn't it, how we always remember how people fell in love?

We rested. The sun began to set. Nancy stood in its golden light, and Nick took her picture. One of my favorite photos of her.

I was too tired to stand and do the same.

"Ready?" Nancy asked.

"As I'll ever be," I said.

We started back up the stairs. About four hundred of them. Nancy gripped my elbow and added a little oomph up each one. Within minutes, I was panting. We stopped often to rest.

One rest at a time.

One step at a time.

One day at a time.

We made it up those steps. It took more than an hour. At the top, I was too tired to walk to the car. Nick had to pull around and hoist me in.

I have been unable to walk right since. I stumble. I cannot lift my legs. When muscle fiber breaks down in healthy people, it repairs itself stronger. That is the biology behind exercise. When muscle breaks down in an ALS patient, it never recovers. It is gone forever.

I left a lot of muscle on those stairs.

"Do you regret it?" Nancy asked me recently.

"No," I said.

And I meant it. I do not regret Wreck Beach, not for a second. Because it was beautiful. A moment I cherish and would not trade.

At my next appointment, I told my physical therapist, Kathy, about the Yukon and the beach. Kathy could see how I had weakened in the time I was gone.

"You need to stop," Kathy said. "The effort of traveling is hurting you."

Too late. Nancy's trip had given me a plan for my year. Within a week of returning, I had booked a trip to Hungary with John. I had decided to return to Cyprus. I had promised a trip to each of my children, knowing I could give them nothing more precious than my time.

Kathy said the same thing after each of those trips. "You're weakening. You should stop."

And each time, I replied the same way: "Not a chance."

California

October

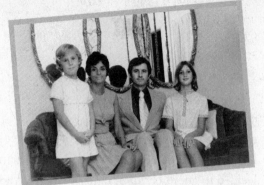

Into the Past

Precious few relationships in my life are like my friendship with Nancy. We've had disagreements, of course, but in thirty years the worst one remains the time in college Nancy copied my outfit to wear to a party.

Nancy and I could have gone to a motel for our trip, and still it would have been special.

It wasn't going to be as easy with others, I knew. Even with John and the kids. And certainly not with my mother, Theodora "Tee" Spencer.

You know when you step out of the shower and have water in your ear? It's not painful. Just bugs ya. And the more you focus on it, the more it bugs ya.

That's the feeling I often had growing up. Like water in the ear. An unease in the soul. Chiefly because of my relationship with Mom.

My mother was a Greek beauty. She had high cheekbones, raven hair, and almond eyes. Her waist was so small you wondered how her organs fit inside. People often told her she looked like Sophia Loren.

Tee's father worshipped her, as did my father. "She was the most exotic, beautiful woman I had ever seen," Dad has said of meeting her.

Soon after their marriage, Mom had a life-threatening miscarriage. And my parents both carried a gene for hemophilia. So they decided to adopt children rather than bear them.

They adopted my sister Stephanie, a beautiful brunette, in 1964.

When they adopted again two years later, Mom requested a child of Greek heritage. One with college-educated parents, she specified on the application. With no red hair and no freckles.

She custom-ordered her ideal child: one like herself.

And there I came. Pudgy. Blond. Beady blue eyes.

The unremarkable-looking daughter of a remarkable beauty.

Most days this was not an issue. As long as I did well in school—and I did very well—Mom was happy. But when Tee was peeved about something, watch out! When her cruel side flared, she hissed things I will never forget:

"My natural child would not do that!"

"My natural child would not look like you!"

"Fat slob!" she often called me. She would puff up her cheeks with air. "This is how you look, you beady-eyed cow."

I was perhaps ten pounds on the heavy side.

Stephanie and I joked often about Mom's disappointment in me, laughing about how "those adoption folks musta pulled a fast one" on her, since I clearly wasn't Greek.

I remember being thrilled when people said I looked like Dad, because he had blue eyes too. I so wanted to resemble somebody. And so wanted to be close to him.

My relationship with Mom changed as I got older and pushed back. I was not scared one whit to say, "Screw you!" Or, "If you lay a hand on me again, I will tell Dad!"

Now, this did not happen on a daily basis, nor even a weekly one. Mom and I might go months without a scene. But when there was one—especially when Tee mocked my looks—it marked me. It left me feeling like a foreign exchange student in my own home.

Our personalities were as different as our looks. Tee shunned attention and was always artificially proper in public. Always smiled and insisted everything was wonderful, even when it wasn't. Honesty made Tee nervous. What would people think?

I was quasi-incorrigible. I set the clocks forward in junior high so we'd go to lunch sooner. I snipped the ends off the teacher's pet's ponytail. I sideswiped the garage after an illicit drive in Dad's Camaro when I was fourteen.

I have scads of pictures of myself with my eyes crossed, puffing out my cheeks, my favorite clown pose. Mom must have hated that.

It wasn't that I was a bad kid, despite the Camaro.

I was a straight-A honor student voted Most Likely to Succeed, a drum major, a class officer, and a member of the homecoming court.

My high school crush, David Hruda, broke my heart when he told me, "You're too nice for a boy like me." And he was right.

But Mom was convinced I was trouble—and that her natural child would not have been.

Then there was religion.

My parents are lifelong members of an enormous Southern Baptist church. Their church is attended by some of the most caring people you'll ever meet. I never received anything but kindness from the members there.

About high school, though, I began to question the Baptists' one-way-to-heaven beliefs. I cringed at the converted Jew they trotted out before the congregation, saying he had found the only way to salvation: "Accept Jesus Christ as your Lord and Savior."

What about the millions of people, I asked, who don't know Jesus? Or don't worship him? The Buddhists? The Muslims? The Taoists? The Hindus? What about the Jews, whose belief system pre-dates Christianity by more than a thousand years?

Millions of people follow ancient belief systems of which Jesus is not a part. "What about them?" I asked.

"They go to hell. So we must save them," was the Baptist answer.

My heart said no. And I left that Baptist church as soon as I was old enough, joking I would only go back there in a pine box.

A truth that hits me more each day.

After high school, I lit out for college far away, at the University of North Carolina in Chapel Hill. I studied abroad in Switzerland. Majored in international studies and interned at the United Nations.

My parents paid for all this, including my extensive travel, even though they never traveled then nor understood my desire to do so.

I became spoiled. I went to Dad after college and proposed that if he financed a trip around the world, I would get a job afterward and pay him back. He said, "Susan, I think you got that backward. Travel is the reward you get after working."

So I spent my twenties divining ways to travel and live abroad. Paid for everything myself. Grew away from my parents in spirit, as well as physical miles.

Even after John and I had children and settled back in south Florida, there was more distance between my parents and us than the mile that separated our homes.

In 2007, two years before I started showing symptoms of ALS, I snuck away to Miami for a weekend with Mom's sisters, Sue and Ramona. The trip was a secret because Tee would have a hissy fit if she knew, scared to death we might talk about her. Those Damianos sisters—who by the way look exactly alike—are forever locked in pettifogging. At times, they have gone years without speaking to one another, in a huff about something or other.

The first thing I said when I got to Miami: "I'm not talking about Tee. And neither are you." Sure enough, it wasn't long before her sisters started in on Tee. And like so many times before, I thought, How the hell did I end up in this bickering clan?

When I returned home, there was a letter in my mailbox. It was from a social worker at the Children's Home Society of Florida. It read: "If you are Susan Spencer born on 12/28/66, please contact me. I have some important information for you."

I knew exactly what it was.

I called the next day. "Yes. That's me. I was adopted through your agency."

"Your birth mother would like to have contact with you," the social worker said.

Now, I've always known I was adopted. Once, as a teen-ager, when things were tense with Tee, I paid to be part of a state registry to unite parents and children if both entered matching information.

Tee was appalled when she found that out.

But after my teenage years, finding my birth parents was never a priority to me. Indeed, on the day I received the let-ter, I had not thought about being adopted in a decade.

I was forty years old with three children of my own. I was happy.

The moment hit me hard.

So hard, I backed away. I put on my journalist's hat, divested myself of emotion, and simply copied down the information about my birth mother. She's a retired nurse. Okay. A gardener. Fine. A racquetball player. Loves to travel. (So that's where I got it!) She had just participated in a three-day walk for breast cancer research. She had a daughter who urged her to find me.

Sounds like a respectable human being, I thought, re-lieved.

"And why did she give the baby up for adoption?" I asked, avoiding the word *me*.

"She would explain it best. Would you like to receive a letter from her?"

"Yes."

I hung up and stared at my notes. I did not cry. I did not

cheer. I did not immediately call anyone to tell them. I just thought: Holy shit!

In the weeks that followed, I panned my life, wondering how I would have reacted at other times. If my birth mother came for me when I was fifteen, I would have said, "Get me outta here!"

At twenty-five: "Why did you do that to me? Why didn't you like me?"

But at forty, after children of my own, the angst was long gone. I knew it wasn't personal, that when she gave me away she did not know me.

I imagined handing my newborns off to a stranger, forever wondering what had happened to them. I realized the emotional toll of adoption was harder on the mother than the child.

I wanted to meet her. I wanted to tell this woman thank you, to assure her that everything had turned out all right.

I wanted to see my face in the face of another adult for the first time in my life.

The letter came inside a manila envelope from the Children's Home Society. I felt the outline of it inside. I smelled it. I put the manila envelope in my car, tucked right by the driver's seat, and drove around for weeks with it there.

I was nervous. Would I like her? Would she like me?

I felt badly for my parents, as if I were betraying them. I thought a better daughter would have said, "No, thank you. I have parents. I want nothing to do with you."

I felt worse for my sister, Stephanie, also adopted. I thought this might wound her, make her wonder why her own birth mother had not looked for her.

I decided that my mother, Tee Spencer, was the only person on the planet I would ever call "Mom." Then, alone one Sunday afternoon, I opened the letter.

In neatly flowing cursive, I read her name: Ellen Swenson. In 1966, she had been a nurse at the Mayo Clinic. He was a doctor. They had a brief fling, and she got pregnant. She moved away and never told him, putting the baby up for adoption as soon as it was born.

There were pictures. One a close head-and-shoulders shot. Ellen was blond, with small blue eyes, a wide white smile. I ran to the bathroom mirror and held the photo beside my face. My breath caught in my throat. I looked like her!

I looked away. The moment was like staring at the sun. So intense, I had to turn away. I had to slow down and let my eyes adjust.

Months later, I wrote Ellen a letter, confirming that I believed she was my birth mother.

"For long tracts of my life I longed to meet you. And just when things settled, when I was overwhelmed with my own children and the longing slipped away, there you came. Life is funny like that. Perfect like that," I wrote.

Initially, I had written back to her as a journalist. As a journalist, if someone tells you an incredible story, by Jove, you investigate. If someone says they're your birth mother, you damn well check the facts. So I did. I wrote and asked Ellen to reveal details of my birth, like the hospital name, that only she and I would know.

She wrote back with all the right answers.

This is the real deal, I thought as I walked around for a week in a daze. This is the real deal. This is the real deal.

Now, I have never been in an earthquake. But I imagine it similar.

A sudden shock rattles your soul. The ground shifts. In minutes it is over, but it takes a long time to find your center of balance again.

So I waited and waited, until I could write her back with my heart.

No hurry, I told myself. The woman waited forty years. She can wait a little longer.

I flung myself into busy. I had three kids, a fifty-hours-a-week job, friends who needed me. Gawd, I have to put the past behind me, I thought. Do I really need this intrusion?

Somewhere in this fog, as I was hurtling through lunch one day, my mother called. My "real" mother, the woman who raised me, Tee Spencer.

I will never forget sitting in the parking lot of the Middle East Bakery, mentioning oh-so-casually that I would like to come by and talk to her and Dad.

"What's wrong!?" Mom said.

"We'll talk in person," I said, wanting to just wolf down my falafel and get off the phone.

"Are you sick?" she asked.

"No. Later, Mom, we'll talk."

"TELL ME!"

"My birth mother contacted me. It's really her."

Silence.

Silence.

Then, in a quivering voice, my mother said: "I knew this day would come. I always knew it would come."

Now, if there is a person to be thrown headlong into an emotional identity crisis with, it is not Tee Spencer. Why? Because she is insecure. Look at her the wrong way, and her feelings get hurt.

"Do you still love us?" she asked.

Oh Gawd, I thought. This is going to be a nightmare.

A few days later, I put copies of the letters between Ellen and me in a manila folder and took them to my parents' house. To be frank, I don't remember what was said. Kinda like when I interviewed famous people. I turned on the recorder and talked on autopilot, listening from a cloud. But that day, I had no recorder.

I do remember the first of Dad's very few questions: "Where does she live?"

"California."

"Good. Far away," he said. "You don't want her just droppin' in."

I remember my mother bringing out the little pink baby dress she brought me home in. And the little yellow one she brought Stephanie home in.

No, I don't remember the words. But I remember the feeling. Isn't that what really matters? How we are left feeling?

I felt sorry for them. Mom's little pink dress. Dad's paralyzed emotion.

I felt guilty. Because I knew in my heart I was going to do what I wanted, and they knew it too. It had always been that way. No guilt nor risk nor fear had ever dissuaded me from doing what I wanted.

It had always been Me, the child they could not control. And Them, the oft-appalled parents.

That meeting slowed me down, though, made me idle a while. I did not act. I went weeks and weeks without writing Ellen back.

Mom asked now and then if I had had further contact with Ellen.

"No."

Then Mom said something that impressed me, and I am one tough cookie to impress. Mom—the woman I was convinced would cower and focus on herself—said: "Don't leave her hanging like that, Susan. She is hurting. She is a mom."

Still, I waited.

I have often in my life been guided by invisible signs. I say, "The gods are divining this," when circumstances allow for something otherwise unlikely.

Like the fact that, after years of trying, I was accepted into a program for journalists at Loyola Law School in Los Angeles that summer. An all-expense-paid trip to California landed in my lap.

The gods had served up the perfect cover story.

"Well, Mom," I told Tee, "if I am already in California, I may as well meet her."

"You do what you want," she said. "We will support you. Just please don't tell your children."

"Okay, Mom, I won't."

So I wrote Ellen the letter. I told her that, yes, she was my birth mother, and that I was coming to California.

Because life, when you least expect it, is perfect like that.

•   •   •

I went to California in June 2008. I am tempted to say this was a year before my ALS, but I don't know if that's true. The ALS could have been with me already, but unnoticeable. It could have been with me always, since the moment of my birth.

Suffice to say, I suspected nothing. I spent a week at the Loyola Law workshop, where the keynote speaker was the lawyer who had just won the court battle overturning the ban there on same-sex marriage. "The world is changing," I kept hearing. "The world is changing."

And the future so unknown.

Afterward, I visited a dear college friend in Los Angeles, Cathy, whom I had roomed with and traveled with while studying in Switzerland. We talked about old times, broke out photos of the Alps and the Hofbrauhaus and Carnevale in Venice.

I thought of all my parents had given me. They had sacrificed so much to launch Stephanie and me to college. I thought of Ellen. My thoughts pinged uncontrollably back and forth.

I have had such a good life. Why am I doing this?

This is part of you.

What will she be like? What if I don't like her?

What if you do like her?

God, I hope she doesn't lock me in a bear hug and start gushing.

If she's anything like you, she won't.

Ellen lived five hours north of Los Angeles, in Sonoma

County. My wine-loving self marveled at my geographic fortune. I was raised by teetotalers, but I have always loved to drink.

A friend hired a driver to take me to Sonoma. Nancy offered to fly out and meet me for the drive. Nancy and I went everywhere together, talked about everything, supported each other through every major life event. This time, I declined. Not wanting any distraction. Wanting to be absolutely alone.

Just me, my thoughts, and Ellen. A onetime meeting. To hear details. Thank her. And leave her behind. That was my plan.

In the end, I opted to ride a crowded bus. Now that I was here, I didn't want to be alone. I put in my iPod earbuds and played one song over and over, Kate Voegele's "Lift Me Up." Her sparrow voice rose and fell in tandem with my heart.

> *This road*
> *is anything but simple.*
> *Twisted like a riddle.*
> *I've seen life and seen love.*
> *So loud*
> *The voices of our mad doubts.*
> *Telling me to pack up and leave town.*

I arrived in Sebastopol and holed up in a hotel a few miles from Ellen's place. I had requested that we not talk beforehand. I'd simply appear at her door at the appointed time the next morning.

I walked halfway to her house, judging the distance,

working off nervous energy. Then I hung around the Sebastopol town square, watching barefoot women with long hair
and tie-dye shirts nurse their children while long-haired men
smoked pot.

I bought dinner at the Whole Foods Market. The store
had an odor of overripe people or overripe food. I ordered a
tofu Reuben (tofu!?) and returned to the square. As I bit into
the rubbery Reuben, the thought dawned on me: Ellen's a
hippie!

How cool.

I gave the rubbery Reuben another bite, hoping the next
one might be better. It wasn't.

A hippie. How . . . cool?

An older man approached me, looking as if he hadn't
changed clothes since the 1970s, and smelling like he hadn't
bathed since then either. He asked me for a cigarette.

My God, I thought, I hope she's not like that.

Now, don't get me wrong. I love the hippie spirit. And
I enjoyed a little Maui Wowie back in college, notably one
hazed-over semester as I lusted after a gorgeous UNC swimmer with a four-foot bong and twenty-gallon lungs.

So yes, I have the heart and soul of a hippie. But the taste
of a woman from Palm Beach. I love BCBG, high heels, nice
jewelry, and good hygiene. I would not be caught dead in a
pair of Birkenstocks or with hairy armpits.

I handed the time traveler a cigarette and my tofu Reuben, still oozing Thousand Island dressing. "You'll enjoy it
much more than me," I told him, heading back to my hotel.

Now, when I get nervous, I get calm. Yes, I know. Makes
no sense, but 'tis true. Before I do a live shot on national tele-

vision, for instance, I consciously slow my breathing and heart rate. Breathe, Susan, breathe, I tell myself, slowing down.

The morning of meeting my birth mother, I passed on the coffee and did just that. I showered, gathered myself, and selected a very plain outfit. Jeans. Black shirt. No jewelry.

Hippies don't like gold chains, I thought.

But, boy, I do!

I slipped my high wedge heels into my bag. Couldn't meet my birth mama in flats, I thought, that just wouldn't be me.

Mom had made Ellen a small photo album, with a picture of me from every year of my childhood, from newborn to college graduate. Tee had taken the time to find special photos for a stranger she was so fearful of.

A precious gift for Ellen, and more so for me. That photo album was the dearest and most surprising thing Mom ever did for me. It was so stunning in its thoughtfulness and care, it overwrote her mistakes of the past.

I took a long look at that album, kissed it, breathed. I slipped it into my bag. I set out walking to Ellen's house.

And immediately felt lonely.

I called Nancy, crying. "I wish you had come," I told her.

"I am at your side in spirit," she said, crying too.

I walked and walked, up a steep incline, out onto a highway lined with apple orchards. I realized I had misjudged the distance. It was miles farther than I thought.

Shit. Shit! I'll be late. She'll worry I'm not coming.

Then that snarky thought pinged again: She waited forty years. She can wait a little longer.

I slowed down, getting my Zen on, staring at the orchards. The trees lined up like soldiers, protecting me. There were brown hills braided with green grapevines. White puffs overhead. It was beautiful.

At the top of Ellen's shady lane, I stopped and slipped out of the present. I pushed aside emotion and became an observer of my own life. As I walked down the short road, I started mentally recording, as if making notes for a newspaper article: bushes, mailbox, trees, sky. I stood at the top of Ellen's driveway, gazing at her small house. It was deep red and kinda looked like a barn. A vast rose garden neatly edged a small patch of green grass.

I put on my high heels, sticking my flats in my bag. As I reached to unhook the latch on the garden gate, I was surprised to see my hand shaking.

The front door stood open, the mesh screen shut. THE QUEEN IS IN, said a sign at the door.

Oh boy, I thought.

The wind chime tinkled.

"Hello?" I called out.

For a minute, nothing, and then there she was, standing on the other side of the screen door. Healthy. Smiling. Casual. Warm.

"Hello. I'm Susan."

"Hello. I'm Ellen."

"Sorry I'm late. I walked. It took me longer than I thought."

"You walked all the way in those shoes?" she said, pointing at my heels.

"No, I have sneakers."

When she heard of my shoe switch, Ellen later told me, she knew I was her daughter.

Ellen opened the screen door, and I stepped inside. She did not hug me. Nor I her. We simply stared at one another, time downshifting into slow motion.

Her eyes. Her small blue eyes. They were mine, just bluer.

Her calves. Her ankles. All my life, people had complimented me on my calves and ankles, and there they were on her.

Her shirt featured three glasses—white wine, red wine, champagne. "Group Therapy," it read. It felt like me.

Ellen asked me to sit down. The sofa was plaid, a folded blanket on the back. Bright yellow walls. A lamp with a pink-fringed shade like you might see in a boudoir. Some modern glass knickknacks. Some Asian-inspired pieces. Books, books, books. And outside, visible through a window, that gorgeous rose garden.

"My mother made something for you," I said, crying, and handed her the photo album.

And just like that, it began. An easing of the soul. A way to a better understanding of my personality. My quirkiness. My directness. My little bit of hippie with a sense of style.

A year later, on our way to Hawaii in the summer of 2009, John and I spent an afternoon with Ellen. So much for thanking my birth mama and leaving her behind. She was a part of my life now. I wanted John to meet her. I wanted to know her better.

We went to a beach park. We took off our shoes. John laughed when he saw our feet side by side, bunions bulging, the same French fry toes. "Now I know you two are related," he said, as he took a picture of Ellen and me from the ankles down.

I told John and Ellen I wanted to write a book. "You should call it 'Bunions in the Sand,' " John said.

I had noticed my withered left hand only a few weeks before. I didn't mention it on that trip, but as I searched for medical answers over the next six months, I realized the serendipity of Ellen appearing when she did.

Ellen came to Florida that year for Thanksgiving. She was visiting her daughter, a crew member on a yacht docked in Fort Lauderdale. (I met her daughter, who was more than ten years younger than me, a few times. Attended her wedding in Seattle. But we've had no contact since then.)

Afterward, Ellen stayed for a few days at a hotel near my house. I had respected my parents' wishes and not told my children about her, but I took them to the hotel, knowing she would like to see them. We swam. We lunched. We took so many pictures Marina asked, "Are you, like, a relative or something?"

"No, I'm just Ellen," she said.

I showed Ellen my hand. I questioned her about her medical history. Neither she, nor any member of her family, had had anything similar.

I cherish that, especially now, above all Ellen's other gifts: the peace of mind, knowing my ALS isn't genetic. My children will inherit many things from me, but they will not inherit my fate.

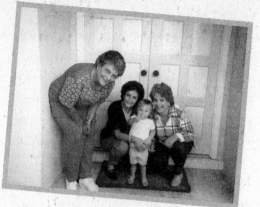

Family Reunion

Mom never talked about Ellen. She didn't ask any meaningful questions about our meeting. She didn't understand Ellen's importance to me, and the relationship hurt her. Tee dealt with that hurt through silence: the kind that says more than words.

Her feelings can be summarized in the question she asked Nancy when I wasn't around, the same one she had asked me months before: "Susan still loves us, doesn't she?"

My feelings crystallized around a short cruise Mom and I took together in February 2011. This was four months before my diagnosis, and a few weeks before my trip to New Orleans with Nancy, when I consciously admitted to myself for the first time that I probably had ALS.

Still deep in denial, I spent the cruise on the ship's pool deck, icy beer bucket beside me, thigh-to-oiled-thigh in the sun-worshipping crowd. The international belly flop contest was on: large, hirsute men from Ohio flung themselves aloft into the pool as I led the sideline vocal scoring.

"Ten!" I'd holler out for the biggest splat of skin.

Mom passed her time in our cabin, struggling to relax. The crowds, the heat, the noise, it was too much for her to handle. She was way, way afield of her comfort zone—the one where she controlled everything.

So she found problems. The ship's housekeeping staff had folded our bath towels into animal shapes. Marina loved the cute monkey. Tee promptly unfolded the monkey so the towel would be ready for her use the next morning.

Tee came to me twice at the pool. Once to announce to the men and women around me that I was married. The second time to remind me that if I did not turn in my towel, I would be charged $20, and she would NOT be paying for it.

We were cruising to the Bahamas to attend Mom's family reunion in Nassau. She had paid the way for me and Marina, a generous gift. But she was drawing the line at towels.

It was a serious family reunion, not one of those barbecue-in-the-park deals. During the next day, we did a walking tour of the old family sites and the graveyard, my legs still strong. Two of our relatives' graves were unmarked. We placed flowers. My parents talked of hiring a stonecutter to mark the graves.

A Greek Orthodox priest gave a history of the faith on the island. Tee's father's family had emigrated from Greece to the Bahamas and Florida. The Damianos clan had been among the seminal Greek Orthodox families in the area.

Even though Tee's mother had raised her Southern Baptist, Tee never lost her Greek heritage. In one of my favorite childhood memories, Mom would tickle me, bury her pointy nose in the corner of my eye, and wiggle it around. Her Greek nose, she called it. Even noses, in memories of my childhood, were Greek.

We returned to the ship to rest before the formal dinner. The day had gone well. We had enjoyed being together.

Then Tee decided she wasn't going to the dinner. I'm not sure why. Perhaps she was tired. More likely someone had said something that peeved her. My dad followed suit. Then Tee's sister, Sue, elected not to go, followed by Sue's daughter and grandson.

It was a seated dinner at the Nassau Yacht Club, which the organizers had gone to great effort and expense planning—a full buffet and bar, a photographer to shoot each branch of the family.

"It's rude not to go," I barked at Tee.

No matter.

Marina stayed behind to hang out with her cousin. I set out alone.

My mother's older sister, Ramona, was there with her daughter and son-in-law, Mona and Mike. Ramona is the matriarch of the family and its biggest cheerleader. She keeps up with cousins near and far. Family means everything to her. And there Ramona sat, at a huge festively decorated table, essentially alone.

At the buffet, I struggled holding the plates. My left hand was near useless, and I had trouble cutting my food. I put down my utensils and looked around the room. I saw the large family pods packed around other tables, laughing and chatting.

I had a few cocktails, which was a bad idea. It made our predominantly empty family table seem sadder.

A speaker recounted our family's Greek heritage. Then the emcee asked people to come to the microphone and share memories.

I wanted to share the story of how I had recently discovered my birth history, which included true-blue Greek ancestry. I wanted to tell them how proud I was to be a Damianos. How much their support and kinship meant to me.

I went to the mike, looked out over the faces, looked at our near-empty family table, and started crying. Bawling, really, in front of the crowd.

Mike sent Ramona to stand by me. A cousin, Flora, also came up to stand by my side. They put their arms around me. I eked out something and sat down, appalled at my public blubbering.

"Greek or not, we'll keep her," Ramona told the crowd.

A few minutes later, thank goodness, a cacophony of whistles, drums, trumpets, and cowbells filled the silence. The surprise of the evening: a Bahamian junkanoo band!

The performers were festooned in feathers and sequins, their headdresses towering over us. They shimmied, bopped, the bass drum *boom-boom-boom*ing, the leader's whistle shrieking to start and stop them parading about the tables. A sinewy young girl performed what I call a booty dance, gyrating her hips just so.

Maybe it's best Tee's not here after all, I thought.

I stepped outside, away from the noise and spectacle. For Tee, the noise and spectacle—especially her daughter's

spectacle—would have been too much. She did not understand how much I was struggling.

The next morning, Mom asked me how the dinner was.

"Very nice," was all I replied.

I suppose I hoped my illness would close the distance between us. That because I was dying, Mom and I would talk.
I wanted to resolve issues from my childhood that poisoned
our relationship.

I wanted to tell her that Ellen changed nothing. That she
was still my mother, and I loved her just the same.

Instead, Mom closed off. After my diagnosis in June, she
did not reach out to me, either for information or to comfort.
She would come by for short visits, always leaving after a few
minutes. The talk got smaller, not bigger. Sometimes, she
barely looked at me.

The door to understanding was closed.

In September, a week after Nancy and I planned the trip
to the Yukon, John and I had a small party. *Dateline* was air-
ing a piece on Dalia Dippolito, a local hottie who'd tried to
hire a hit man to whack her hubby. I was one of the featured
experts, as I had covered her trial extensively in the spring.
I had filmed my *Dateline* segment the day after my ALS diagnosis.

"With me," I told the producer, joking about my slowed
speech, "you won't have to worry about filling an hour."

Mom was excited: she loved to call all her friends when I
was on TV. She wasn't coming to the party, but she offered
to make her delicious Greek salad, with olives, feta, and her
special homemade dressing.

As she handed the salad to me that afternoon, I noticed that the whites of her eyes seemed yellow. I started to say something, but in that moment someone called to ask directions, or Marina asked if she could go to a friend's house instead of hanging out with adults, or Wesley asked out of the blue, "Who's your favorite character in *Lilo & Stitch*?"

When I turned back, Mom was gone.

I got a call from Dad two days later. "We're at the emergency room," he said. "Mom is jaundiced and vomiting."

I zipped straight there. Mom was lying in an examining room with a little throw-up vessel handy. She was dressed in a red shirt, jeans, and . . . yellow.

Her eyes. Her face. Even her hands were yellow.

You have to understand, a week before, Mom seemed in perfect health. Even at seventy-one, she walked miles each day. She knew most of the residents on her route, she had done it so long and so often. She led an exercise class at her church. She ate healthy, didn't drink, and absolutely never smoked a cigarette.

She was the cleanest-living person I knew. You had to cajole her to take a Tylenol for a headache. Mom was so healthy, in fact, she didn't even have a doctor.

Jaundice is usually associated with a liver problem. Mom had never drunk alcohol or engaged in any remotely risky behavior, so her problem must not be a big deal, right?

"There's something pressing on her bile duct," Dad told me. "Something on her pancreas. That's what's making her jaundiced."

"Is it pancreatic cancer?" I blurted out.

"I don't know. I hope not," Dad said, steely as ever.

The doctors told us the only way to know was to remove the growth immediately. The surgery nearly killed her—twice. From that moment until four months later, my mother never left a hospital or medical facility.

There were times in the intensive care unit when things were so grave, we scurried to her side in the middle of the night. Times when I held my iPhone up to her ear and played her favorite hymn, "Holy Ground," convinced she would die that day.

At one point, Stephanie, Dad, and I talked of planning a memorial. "I want a Celebration of Life, not a funeral," Dad said.

Stephanie still says the saddest thing she's ever seen was me hobbling down the hospital corridor on my weakening legs, trying to reach Mom before she bled out and died.

Mom survived. A miracle to the few, like me, who saw her on the ventilator, unable to breathe on her own.

It was brutal. A time of stress and worry. Of fearing the worst. I would spend whole weeks unable to sleep and days without food.

It was a time also of reflection, for being at the bedside of an extremely ill loved one, when you are extremely ill, stirs thoughts. I saw myself on that bed, with the tubes, the ventilator to breathe for me, the distraught loved ones. When we had to make hard decisions, Dad had no idea what Mom wanted. She had certainly never discussed anything with Stephanie or me.

I decided not to drag my family through that. To plot everything out, with specifics. Medical orders. Hospice. Living will. "I don't want a feeding tube," I told John after seeing and smelling Mom's. "I don't want to be kept alive when the doctors say the humane things to do is let me go."

It was also a time of devotion. Of togetherness with Dad and Steph, who were constantly at Mom's side. In his grief, Dad spoke to Steph and me more than ever before. We held our own family reunion, right there at Mom's side.

Those days reminded me how lucky I was to have a family. I felt their love and drew strength from it. These were the people who had always been with me.

And Tee was a part of that. She was my mother. At her bedside, I felt a closeness to her I hadn't felt in a long time. I realized how much she meant to me, as it devastated me to see her suffer so.

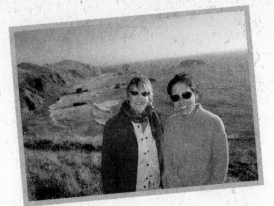

The Yurt

My trip with Nancy to the Yukon was scheduled for October, about a month after Mom was hospitalized. The trip of a lifetime, but I almost didn't go. Mom's condition was critical as the date approached. I couldn't leave her.

Then Mom improved. She stabilized and gave me the okay. She wanted me to experience the wonder of the northern lights, and she knew how much Nancy meant to me.

I never told her I was making another stop on the way.

There were no direct flights from south Florida to Vancouver, where we would catch a plane to the Arctic. When I realized that, I scheduled the layover for San Francisco. Nancy and I would visit Ellen, then continue on to Canada.

I kept that part of the trip a secret from my parents. It would have been too complicated to explain, and I didn't want to cause Mom pain.

Now, Nancy and I had decided that on this trip there

would be no skimping. "Life's too short to stay in crappy ho-tels," I said. We booked the Four Seasons in Vancouver. And we rented a town car and driver to tour San Francisco before heading to Ellen's house, an hour away.

Our driver was named Irving. He wore a black suit and black chauffeur cap, but looked barely old enough to drive. He assured us, though, he had been chauffeuring around the Bay Area for years. And he had a GPS.

The three of us bopped around San Francisco: took a tour of the Bay, had an Irish coffee at the Buena Vista Cafe, went to Chinatown.

We turned a corner and caught sight of a rocky island in an azure bay. "Wow! Is that Alcatraz?" Nancy asked.

"I don't know," Irving said.

I had heard of these creatures: young people who have grown up with GPS and have no sense of place or direction without it. Who never see the world around them, only the screen. But not recognizing Alcatraz after years in San Fran? Ridiculous!

Nancy had her sights on dinner at a certain restaurant in Chinatown, recommended by a friend. Miss Google-vision rarely forgets a meal (or misses one). She can recall years later the crispy parsnips sprinkled on the ricotta-and-spinach ravi-oli in butter sage sauce. And woe to the soul who interrupts her daily gastronomic pas de deux.

I was envisioning a repeat of my last meal in Chinatown—dim sum, ceremoniously served, steamer baskets and plates of bite-size delicacies covering the white linen table.

Sam Wo was not that place.

For starters, the entrance was a kitchen door propped

open. A colander full of entrails draining was our first sight.

The cooks shooed us past the steaming woks to a dark stairwell. Nancy helped me up the stairs into the dining room, which looked as if it belonged on a ship. A Viking ship. The ceilings were low and the tables utilitarian blocks with benches. A dumbwaiter lined with newspaper brought food up from the kitchen.

"Let's just order something fun," I said.

So we did. Singapore Style Chow Mai Fun. It was $5.25. Nancy's friend had led us to the cheapest dump in Chinatown.

I don't remember the Sam Wo food being good, bad, or otherwise. No, I blotted from my mind the fact that I ate there right after using Sam Wo's bathroom. Nancy took pictures, it was so dirty. Dust so thick on the exhaust fan you could braid it. A white sink with just one ungrimed area where the water and soap hit.

"That was an adventure!" I said as I returned to the table.

We would chuckle over and over about our Sam Wo experience. And we were not a whit surprised to learn months later that the health department had shut down the restaurant, citing a host of fire and sanitation code violations. Including rodent feces in the kitchen.

Our chauffeur Irving picked us up at the kitchen door. We drove over the Golden Gate bridge at sunset, stopping for a photo. There was a bride doing the same, freezing in her strapless gown.

I had told Nancy to pack only one carry-on bag for the trip, hoping to travel light. Which Nancy did. Then I pulled up with two suitcases overstuffed with full-length cashmere coats and more sweaters than there were days on the trip.

I couldn't roll the heavy suitcases with my weakened arms, so Nancy did the lugging. "Whaddaya got in here?" she asked. "A piano?"

"No. Two boot sets. Two coats. Six cashmere sweaters."

So we were stylin' in our chauffeured black town car and cashmere when we pulled into hippie headquarters—the Sebastopol town square.

We were early, so we parked to kill some time, bought a German chocolate cake to take to Ellen and hot tea to sip on the square.

At this time, there were demonstrations going on called "Occupy [Insert Name of City Here]." An international protest movement against social and economic inequality, people camping out in cities around the world.

There was an "Occupy Sebastopol" under way. We sat nearby, enthused to see the social activism, talking of how if we were younger we might have joined in. Laughing at ourselves. The men nearby thought we were laughing at them.

"Ack! We look like capitalist pigs. Let's go. Where's Irving?"

Ellen's home is surrounded by an extraordinary garden with eighty-five varieties of roses. The setting is secluded and cool; the breeze sweeps through her home, tinkling wind chimes all around. She set us up in an airy bedroom, asking only that we close the shutters during the day to keep sunlight from fading the family quilt on a wall.

Ellen loved her childhood on a farm in Iowa, where they didn't have indoor plumbing until she was seven and electricity until she was fourteen. "Idyllic," she said. There were mementos, like the quilt, all around.

She left the farm for adventure. She studied nursing in Minnesota. Took a bus, while pregnant, to California, then cross-country to Florida. After giving me up for adoption, she continued nursing—including in and around Haight-Ashbury, the San Francisco 'hood where drug culture and psychedelic rock flourished.

Ellen was indeed a hippie, she said, but she never "checked out." Always maintained a job. Retired from years of training nursing students to work with psychiatric patients.

As Nancy pointed out, Hollywood could not script two more opposite women than Ellen and Mom.

A hippie and a Baptist.

An adventurous experimenter and a devoted housewife. I doubt Mom knew anything about drugs.

Mom wanted more than housewife-hood for Stephanie and me. She wanted us to have choices, and she drove us hard to succeed. Mom was an academic taskmaster. Sweated each low test grade. REQUIRED straight A's.

She never made us wash dishes. "It's more important that you study," she'd say, washing the dishes herself.

And it worked. Both Steph and I were top students in high school and entered fine universities.

My first semester of college—my first time away from Mom—I went wild. The first night, I drank so much spiked fruit punch I hurled red for hours. Then I fell for that UNC swimmer and his four-foot bong. I squeaked by my classes with C's.

The second year I lived with Nancy, the consummate student. She completed projects months before they were due, always earning A's. She urged me to go to the library rather than frat parties and helped keep me straight. With her help, I made my best grades since Mom.

I have always needed someone like that to help rein in my wild side.

Ellen, it soon became apparent, may not have been that person.

I had brought my adoption records, and we discussed them one night. Ellen read the comments on each page, remarking over and over how they were "free of judgment, free of judgment." Amazed. Thankful. Ellen, I realized, was fearful of being judged for what she had done.

It was heavy stuff. Tense. Emotional. I needed a cigarette, but I was out. So I asked Ellen if she had one.

"No," she replied.

To lighten the mood, Ms. Phi Beta Kappa joked: "How about some pot?"

Ellen perked up. "No. But I have a friend who has some."

She called her friend, and we drove over to pick it up. I asked if we needed to pay. "No, no. I did her a big favor. She owes me," Ellen said.

Back at Ellen's house, she got out her pot paraphernalia box. Rolling papers. Pipes. Little one-hit wonders.

"Some of this is my daughter's," Ellen said.

Nancy gave me the can-you-imagine-doing-this-with-Tee? look.

We smoked up. We laughed and laughed. Nancy and I helped Ellen sort through a host of old coats. She tried them on for us, and we gently reminded her of the decade in which they had gone out of style.

Lying in bed that night, I had an epiphany. Mom's hard hand had made me the successful person I was today. My work ethic and self-reliance: those were gifts from Tee.

"Man," I said to Nancy. "I am glad Ellen didn't raise me. Can you imagine me with a pot-smoking mom? I'd have ended up barefoot, stoned, and living in a yurt."

Living in a yurt. Nancy and I have laughed about that phrase ever since.

The next day, Ellen took us to the Sonoma coastline to Goat Rock Beach. To high hills overlooking the Pacific Ocean. There's a massive stone outcrop just offshore. Goats once lived upon it, thus the beach's name.

There are vistas there where you can stare in wonder at miles of craggy coastline and wide beaches. We walked the overlooks. We took pictures.

California sits upon fault lines, where Earth's tectonic plates crash constantly into one another. Throwing up these rocks and cliffs, reshaping entire continents a millimeter at a time. The football stadium at the University of California at Berkeley, which sits directly upon a fault line, is being split apart by this stealthy force. Fourteen inches apart, to be precise, since being built in 1922.

I had once told Ellen that finding her had been like an earthquake. That I would need time to shake off the shock and find balance again.

I felt balance there at the coastline after my stoned epiphany. I felt balance between the dynamic woman who made my body and soul, and the devoted mother who reared me, controlled me, and shaped me.

As we left Goat Rock, I stared at the trees along the highway. Windswept cypress, their branches all pointing the same direction, whipped into form by invisible forces.

Forces still at work today. Shaping continents. Coastlines. The human soul.

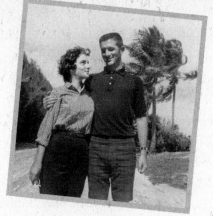

Closing the Loop

In California, Ellen explained the pregnancy to me simply. That it was a sexual fling and nothing more. That the man, Panos Kelalis, was a playboy, and she saw no future with him. That he was intent on returning to his home country of Cyprus, and giving the baby up for adoption seemed the only way out.

Ellen talked of how she plowed through the pregnancy with no emotion. How she told none of her family. How she ran off to Florida and worked as a surgical nurse so no patient was awake to ask her about the baby.

They put her to sleep for my birth, so she would have no memory of it. Against the advice of the adoption workers, Ellen asked to see the baby—to see me—in the nursery, knowing she was having no emotional reaction.

And still she felt nothing.

Wow, that's cold! I thought when I first heard her say that.

Wow, that's strong! I tend to think now.

Ellen acknowledged that as a nurse she understood abortion and could have found a medical colleague to do it. In fact, she later aborted a second unplanned pregnancy. "I have no idea why I never considered it," she said.

I told Ellen I understood her decisions.

To have the baby.

To leave me behind.

If I got pregnant by some man I had zip-zero connection with, and I would have to move someplace I didn't know and never wanted to live in . . . say, a one-stoplight farm town in North Dakota . . . well, I wouldn't go either.

Which is to say I might consider the exact same thing.

Consider, yes, but Ellen did one thing I could not abide: she didn't tell the father.

Panos never knew he had a daughter.

I would have told the father. I would have done it in fairness to him and the child. For I was taught a deep sense of conscience by the two extraordinary people who raised me. My mom and dad.

For years, Dad volunteered at a nursery for AIDS babies. He donated medicine from his pharmacy and went every Wednesday night to hold the babies and rock them. He lived for two years in Ethiopia as a missionary. He started a puppet ministry, hand-making eight hundred puppets on a sewing machine, so that he could share with children the story of Jesus Christ.

I have been frustrated since my illness by Dad's lack of warmth. He is a great man, a caring soul, but he has not spoken to me of ALS. When I told him recently I was signing up for hospice, he said, "Oh." Then changed the subject.

I know he hurts. I have heard him say, when he thought I couldn't hear, "I don't cry, because if I start, I will never stop."

I thought of that, when going over this section in my mind. I thought of how Dad couldn't say those words to me.

But how his actions speak volumes.

How all our actions speak more than we can know.

I thought of how, in a moment, without even stopping to think, Dad rattled off ten feature newspaper articles I had written, even though he had never spoken to me about them. Ten or fifteen years later, he knew the titles. He knew the details. He talked of how I had gathered the information. He remembered the methods I had used.

I wanted, in this last year, to close the loop with Mom and Dad. To heal the rift that had formed as I explored my birth parents, something that did not diminish my love for them.

I understand now that that moment will not occur. We will not talk our way to understanding. It's just not in their natures.

And as ALS reminds me each day, you can't fight nature.

Rather, I embrace the small things. Like the words of a friend who talked to Mom and Dad the day after an article about my illness and book deal appeared in the newspaper.

The friend had been mentioned, so Mom went to get him the article. She had fifteen copies of the newspaper, in a neat stack in a cabinet.

"Give this to your mother," she said, handing him one.

Not to just anyone: to your mother.

Because your mother is the person who loves you. Who

has always loved you. Who is proud of you, even if she keeps those feelings locked away in a drawer.

I took many journeys over the course of the year with the people I love. I never even considered a journey with Mom.

Rather, I traveled three thousand miles to California and found peace with the person who had been one mile away all along.

Christmas

December–January

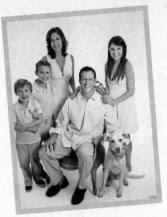

Together

I n November, after I returned from California and the Yukon, I sent an e-mail to my bosses at the *Palm Beach Post*. It read in part:

It's now been three months since I [took a medical leave] from the paper and the job I loved.

It was a privilege to go to work each day and grow democracy, to ferret out stories no one wanted told, to be trusted to inform and, yes, entertain our readers. When someone would ask me: "Who sent you?" I loved to reply: "Well, ma'am, that would be Thomas Jefferson." I so wanted to evolve with the paper and work to keep it a central force in our community . . .

[But now] each day I get weaker. My speech is slurred and my hands so weak I cannot type with any speed . . . I am unable to scurry round, fire off web feeds, and talk without strangers wondering if I'm drunk. I tell you this so you know I am no longer the sturdy, speedy workhorse you need on the breaking news courts beat. Ergo, I resign my position. Four words I type while weeping.

The *Palm Beach Post* kindly offered me any writing assignments I wished, on a freelance basis. I told them I wanted to write personal stories. I wanted to write about learning to embrace life despite illness.

Writing was something I had planned to do all along, a part of living with purpose and joy. Then Mom got sick and life intervened. But with the job officially behind me, and Mom seemingly on the mend, I settled into the holiday season with free time and a plan. I would write about life with ALS. And I would make this Christmas a memorable one.

In years past, with no vacation days left, I often worked through the holidays. With our busy schedules, John and I at times decided it was too much trouble to get out the trove of decorations stashed high in our garage in large bins.

Rather, we'd buy a small tree and make popcorn garlands and construction paper chains with the kids.

This year, I went all out. For days, the kids and I worked slowly through the Christmas bins, opening hundreds of decorations, breaking out the entire Christmas village my aunt Beth had given us piece by piece over years.

We placed red-letter blocks on shelves spelling out words like R-E-J-O-I-C-E and P-E-A-C-E. We hung the children's Christmas crafts and hauled out every Santa, including the Santa toilet seat cover my zany cousin Mona had given us. Marina was such a help, taking over for my fumbling hands.

I don't believe in lots of gifts, but rather giving each child one nice thing. This year, I bought them each a laptop. Marina wrapped them, as well as all the presents for our relatives and friends.

As a gift to ourselves, John and I went to the bank with my life insurance money and paid off our mortgage. John had wanted to invest the money, but I insisted on leaving my family debt-free. I wanted to know that, no matter what, my children would never lose their home.

We returned from the bank to find that home in disarray. And the Christmas letter blocks rearranged by Marina to spell P-E-N-I-S.

Usually, the kids were pretty good at practical jokes. We still laugh about one April Fools' Day, when I hurried in from work in my usual way, hands full of files, probably on my phone yammering away with an editor.

"Have a chocolate!" Marina said, popping one in my mouth. I bit down. It was a chocolate-covered radish.

"Blech!" I said as I spit it out in the kitchen sink.

I flipped on the faucet to rinse my mouth. Marina and Aubrey had taped the sprayer handle in the on position. The spray shot directly in my face, soaking me.

"Hardy-har-har," I said to the chuckling peanut gallery.

I went back to my bathroom. The kids tried to follow me, but I shut the door and sat down on the toilet seat. Which they had coated with nonstick cooking spray.

"Hee, hee, hee," I heard from behind the door.

"Ya got me!" I said, laughing.

I kicked off my heels and put on my comfy pair of leather flip-flops. Which had been slathered inside with marshmallow creme.

Four gags in a row, one after the other.

"Someone's gettin' a whuppin'," I said to the giggle-fitters, which only made us all laugh harder.

This time, though, the Christmas creativity was not so perfect, and I'm not just talking about the P.E.N.I.S. blocks. John and I walked in the door high on our financial milestone to find a white powder mess in the living room. I mean, powder everywhere: carpet, furniture, walls, books.

Marina, fully into the Christmas season, had tried to decorate the tree with a mixture of flour and salt. She thought it would look like snow.

"I read it on the Internet!" she said in response to our stares. Pause. "It didn't work."

John was irate, though he laughs about it now. He cursed as he hauled the tree outside to vacuum it.

A year before, I would've cursed too, because a full day of cleaning needed to be done. But serious illness changes you.

Or simply reveals who you are.

I laughed at the flour fiasco.

No bother. Holidays meant togetherness, with all its messes.

Mom was still in the hospital, so I brought a small tree for her room. Against Dad's wishes—he said hospitals don't want things stuck on the walls—Steph and I decorated Mom's space with hundreds of get-well and Christmas cards she had received. We gave Mom a tablet computer, hoping Dad could get her interested in a book to fill the never-ending hours in the hospital. It was a flop.

On Christmas morning, the *Palm Beach Post* published my first article on ALS. It was the story of my Yukon trip with

Nancy, under the headline: "Among the Northern Lights: Two Life-Long Friends, One Adventure of a Lifetime."

As Nancy's present, I had a copy of the article professionally mounted for her. She gave me a mounted wall hanging of a glorious green aurora. Right away, I hung it at the center of my living room wall.

The year before, John's coworker had given us a CD of Christmas songs. Despite the worsening condition of my left arm, John and I danced slowly around the house that year to the sounds of the season, loosening up for a merengue number, slowing to appreciate Andrea Bocelli's soaring version of "O Come All Ye Faithful."

Then I fulfilled a long-standing wish to serve a Christmas goose, just like in Charles Dickens's *Christmas Carol*. John and I had spent all day preparing the sides and tangerine-rind basting sauce, then roasting the bird.

This year, I had no muscles for dancing, and no strength for slicing, dicing, or handling hot pans.

So on Christmas Eve, a former colleague from the *Post*, Jan Norris, brought a complete Christmas meal. Jan, I would learn in the coming months, had the heart of an angel and—bonus!—was the *Post*'s former food editor.

She brought a feast, everything from a bacon-wrapped date appetizer to a traditional Christmas turkey to a full range of desserts. The goose had been one our tastiest holiday meals, but it's a distant second in my heart to the food Jan prepared for us, despite having her own family to care for on the most special eve of the year.

We ate it on a quiet Christmas afternoon, the kids busy with their new laptops, the torn wrapping paper thrown away. I think it was the first year Wesley enjoyed his gift more than the box and wrapping it had come in.

I do not send Christmas cards, as we have a host of friends who do not celebrate the holiday. Instead I send New Year's cards, celebrating the new beginning we all share. In 2010, our card's message spoke of strengthening our friendship and bodies.

This year, it was about acceptance. The card featured a portrait of our family, taken in the summer, with our dog Gracie sitting beside John, and Wesley holding his stuffed Piglet. It was a bucket-list item, a last family portrait before my cheeks shrank, my body withered, and I stopped looking like myself. Only my left hand, resting on John's shoulder, showed clear signs of ALS.

On the back, I put a quotation from *The Prophet* by Kahlil Gibran. It read:

> *Then the woman said, Speak to us of Joy and Sorrow. And*
>   *he answered:*
> *Your joy is your sorrow unmasked.*
> *And the selfsame well from which your laughter rises was*
>   *oftentimes filled with your tears.*
> *And how else can it be?*
> *The deeper sorrow carves into your being, the more joy you*
>   *can contain.*
> *Is not the cup that holds your wine the very cup that was*
>   *burned in the potter's oven?*
> *And is not the lute that soothes your spirit the very wood that*
>   *was hollowed with knives?*
> *When you are joyous, look deep into your heart and you shall*

*find it is only that which has given you sorrow that is
giving you joy.*

It was an acknowledgment of my illness without mentioning it. A testament to the year I was trying to live.

"It's beautiful," a friend said. "But I don't get it. What
does it mean?"

"It means search your soul for strength," I replied.

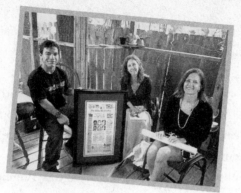

The Party

In early January, my colleagues at the *Post* threw me a going-away party. I had taken my medical leave in August without telling anyone what was wrong. I didn't even tell my colleagues I was leaving. I walked in on a Saturday, when almost no one was around, with the intention of clearing out my cubicle unnoticed.

Too painful. I left everything exactly where it was: my awards in the drawer, my brown sweater hanging on the back of my chair, my map of the cosmos and my children's artwork on my big cork display board.

Five months later, seeing my old colleagues hurt, but not as much.

We gathered at the house of reporter Jane Musgrave. I could not eat and talk at the same time, so I chose conversation. We talked about our years at the *Post* as old veterans talk about a war: hard days, but the best of our lives.

I was reminded of the time, about ten years before, when

I was mugged at gunpoint. For two minutes, I stood face-to-face with three black teens. As a veteran crime journalist, I knew to study features and look for identifying marks. And yet, half an hour later, I realized I couldn't look at suspect mug shots and pick any of them out. Not with any confidence I wasn't fingering an innocent person.

That got me thinking. And thinking led to discovering that eyewitness misidentification is the leading cause of wrongful conviction. Almost 75 percent of prisoners exonerated by DNA had been wrongly identified by an eyewitness.

In 2006, I started writing about eyewitness identification. I wrote extensively of a case where a man received a forty-three-year prison sentence after being identified by a single witness as the shooter in a road rage incident. Vishnu Persad, though, was a different race than originally described and had an alibi: he was across town in a chemistry study group at the time of the shooting.

After five years in prison, his conviction was overturned.

I researched the story of a man arrested for second-degree murder in a bar fight, though he had clear evidence he was hunting in Georgia at the time of the drunken melee.

In another case, a man named Julio Gomez spent five months in jail awaiting trial for murder, even though he lived five counties away. He was the wrong Julio Gomez, and looked nothing like the real killer. Yet an eyewitness had picked him out of a lineup and signed under his picture: "This is the Julio who I witness involved in the murder."

I wrote of three local criminal defense attorneys, all black, who had been misidentified at trial by witnesses. When asked to identify the criminal—the person in danger of being put in jail for a long time—three witnesses at different trials had pointed to the attorney, not his client.

One attorney had been misidentified that way in two separate trials.

My purpose was not to denigrate victims. I felt for them, many suffering years after the crimes. They weren't to blame. And neither were police and prosecutors, who acted in the interest of fairness and were rarely wrong.

But rarely isn't never, and the system had a blind spot. Even the best system in the world, as one of the misidentified attorneys told me, can get "lazy" in enacting change.

And Florida was one of the worst. A decade before, the Department of Justice had released national recommendations on decreasing misidentifications. Police in my county of Palm Beach, and many others in the state, had not adopted them, even though an eyewitness's memory is evidence and should be lifted as carefully as a fingerprint.

My research on eyewitness identification culminated with a front-page article published in January 2011—only weeks before I admitted to myself I had ALS. I had pored over the policies of thirty-two law enforcement agencies. Just three had in place best-practice procedures for creating fair photo lineups, advising eyewitnesses, and documenting identifications.

Within a month, on the recommendation of a statewide panel, the Palm Beach sheriff's office announced it was changing its policies for eyewitness identification. A year later, most of those policies had been written into state law.

"You did that," my friend Nancy said recently. "You helped make the system better."

I disagree. I didn't change the system. Dedicated law enforcement professionals did that. But by highlighting problems, I helped bring the discussion forward, and that made a difference. If not, what purpose does journalism serve?

At the party, my colleagues gave me framed copies of two of those articles. Jane Smith, another *Post* veteran, pointed out that the newspaper used to give Rolex watches to long-time employees on their retirement. No more.

So my colleagues had pitched in and bought me a gift: a 32-gig iPad, top of the line, engraved like those gold Rolexes had once been. It said: "To Susan Spencer-Wendel. From current and former *Post*ies."

So much money was donated, they also gave me iTunes cards.

"I felt like George Bailey at the end of 'It's a Wonderful Life,' " Jane Smith wrote in her note, referring to the scene where people keep spontaneously giving Jimmy Stewart's character money. Jane received so many contributions, she finally told people to stop.

"You see, Susan," she wrote, "you touched so many lives that we got a touch-screen iPad for you!"

For months, that iPad was my constant companion. In December, while working on the story of my Yukon trip with Nancy, I had lost the ability to use a standard computer keyboard. The keys were too far apart and difficult to press.

But I could hunt-and-peck on the iPad touchscreen. I could write again.

I could read books again, even though I could no longer

hold the real ones. I was so excited, I downloaded the entire *Fifty Shades of Grey* trilogy in a minute, thinking I would lap up the bondage scenes. Instead, I soon tired of reading descriptions of juvenile orgasm over and over.

Ah well, sometimes the details disappoint. Smile.

But friendship rarely does.

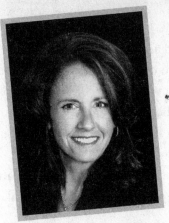

A Gift to Myself

After the party, with kids back in school and John back at work, I gave myself another gift. One based more on want than necessity: permanent makeup.

I love fashion, always have and always will. I was no beauty queen, but I always prided myself on being well put together. Perhaps a form-fitting black dress—not too tight or too short for work. And black heels, four inches, closed toe, a thick heel to signal "not stripper shoes."

Ah, heels, love them. Wore them every day of my adult life, even nine months pregnant. With bunions. Then my legs became too weak. Out went the high heels.

No way was I letting that happen with makeup.

Makeup was my friend. It opened my beady eyes, created cheekbones where none existed, transformed my gullet gateway into kissable lips.

Makeup is precise, an art of millimeters. Fine lines erased around eyes, shadows—sometimes three shades—applied just so on eyelids and under brows, with a dot of sparkly white on the brow bone to open the eyes and make a twinkle.

Like so many women, I had spent scads of money finding the just-so combo for my face. Found a lip color I loved—Raisin Rage—a shade of plum that looked natural and nice. Wore it every day.

Lined my beady eyes to open them up, careful not to draw the line too close to the center, which makes the eyes look closer together.

Brushed multiple coats of mascara on my lashes. I owned three different colors—Very Black, Black, and Brownish Black—plus their waterproof versions.

Even as my hands weakened, I applied makeup. When my fingers curled, I twisted open bottles with my teeth. My magic tubes had chew marks on their sides.

Finally, I gave up closing things—too hard to reopen. I drove around with an open tube of Raisin Rage poised for application, propped in the center console of my car. That worked until the heat came. Then I had a molten plum mess.

My hand began to shake so much I could no longer line my eyes. The mascara wand quivered, so I ended up with more Brownish Black on my eyelid than on my eyelashes.

Failure was not an option. Me without makeup was NOT an option.

Vanity, thy name is Susan.

And I am claiming you. Caring about how you look is not shallow. Pride is the engine of self-respect. Nothing important ever was accomplished by letting the little things slip.

Besides, without makeup, I looked like I had not slept in a decade.

And John putting it on me? Never even entered the realm of possibility.

So I gave myself a late Christmas present: permanent makeup. A euphemism for: tattoo your face. Yes, that is how vain I am. I didn't think twice about needling ink into my eye sockets and lips.

I Googled away. A site advertising "wake up with makeup" caught my beady eye. The artist, Lisa, was a certified micropigmentation specialist. Yes, it's real. Lisa worked in a plastic surgeon's office, where they might tattoo an areola on a new breast after a mastectomy or eyebrows on an accident victim's face.

And she had worked on disabled people like me.

I called. Lisa said something right away that gave me confidence: "I refuse to tattoo anything unusual or that will look bad." Women often asked her to tattoo mole beauty marks on their faces. She declines, she said, because they fade and look blotchy.

Lisa offered tattooing of the eyebrows, eyes, and lips. I signed up for all three.

"Oh, gosh, honey, are you sure?" Steph, also a makeup maven, said. "It's permanent. And painful."

"And my only option," I said.

Pain was not an issue for me. I have a high tolerance for pain. Pregnant in high heels, that was me. I have subjected myself to the most painful body maintenance women can elect to do: the Brazilian bikini wax. After that hair-ripping horror show, pain was not a problem.

"Well, I am definitely going with you," Steph said. "To make sure her tools are clean and she doesn't turn you into a clown."

It takes hours to tattoo a face. Brows, for example, are

drawn one hair at a time, underneath a high-power magnifying glass. Lips take hundreds of pinpricks, each injecting a dot of color under the skin.

But oh, what color? That was the hardest part.

Lisa had custom-ordered a color she thought would work on my lips. She put some on me. It looked like orange Vaseline.

"You won't see that much orange," Lisa said. Permanent ink, she assured me, looks vastly different under the skin.

"No way," I said. "No orange!"

She tried a red. Now, I love red, but only at night.

I asked her to re-create Raisin Rage. She mixed up a plum, which I liked. We selected browns for the eyeliner and brows.

Lisa plucked my brows, then drew on the shape I wanted to add.

Heaven! I thought happily. I'll finally have arches! All my life, I had had skewer-straight brows.

Lisa numbed the area with a cream. She turned on the needle tool.

Zzzz . . . zzzz . . . zzzz, it sounded each time it injected color.

I held my breath for the first ten minutes. Steph watched each stroke. The brown brow color looked purple. Steph asked if that was normal.

"Yes," Lisa said. "Don't worry."

She *zzz, zzz, zzz*ed for an hour on each brow.

She held a mirror up for me to see. My brows looked swollen and bloody, but otherwise fine.

Next came the eyes, open as she *zzz*ed a line flush with my lashes.

"I'd need a sedative for that," Steph said.

I could not flinch. I could not move a hair with the needle so near my eye. I lay still as stone, a deep calm coming over me.

Get your Zen on, Susan.

We decided to add a wee flourish on the outside corners, like an extra-thick lash at the end. A makeup trick that makes eyes look larger and more open.

Lips were last. Lisa warned they would be the most painful and slathered numbing cream all over.

I wanted the entire lip colored, not just lined. Lipstick that has worn away, revealing just lipliner, has always looked ridiculous to me.

Lisa started *zzz-zzz-zzz*ing. I flinched. Lips are sensitive. Why else is a kiss so enchanting?

The wee dip in the center of the top lip is called a Cupid's bow. It felt like Cupid's bow was stabbing me as Lisa worked. I wanted to jump out of my sensitive skin.

I took a deep breath and thought of the most perfect kiss I ever had: a first kiss of intense ardor, yet not too hard, on lips just the right size, touching every millimeter of mine, the soft point of his tongue tracing the outline of my mouth.

I thought and thought of that kiss, that night so many years ago.

And then my lips were done.

I looked in the mirror. Swollen and bloody.

"The appearance will change in the coming weeks," Lisa emphasized for the twentieth time. "The true color comes only after the skin has shed."

She gave me an information sheet on what, when, where, including phases where the tattoos appear blue as skin sheds, or colors disappear altogether, or brows appear markedly larger and darker as they cure.

"Don't worry. It's going to be beautiful!" she said.

Steph and I got in the car for the drive home. I took a look in the rearview mirror. Groucho Marx stared back at me. My brows were big black slugs stuck on my forehead.

I did not look again, just hoped for the best. What's done is done, I thought. No sense in worrying.

Over the next few weeks, my face went psychedelic. I held my breath and religiously put on the healing ointment Lisa recommended and waited, checking off phases on my info sheet.

"How's it look?" I asked John, my husband of twenty years.

Poor guy.

I not only looked like Groucho Marx, I was also a Groucho. What in heaven's name was my husband of twenty years supposed to say?

"Let me put that ointment on so it heals faster," he said.

Good answer.

As my body withered and my looks changed, John always had a good answer. He stuck with me without a word, even when my face was blotchy.

And then the makeup cured. It looked good. Far better than no makeup at all.

It was me, the way I had presented myself to the world for twenty years. Thinner in the cheeks. Less muscle control. But me.

Ah, makeup. Still mine to control.

A part of my body that will remain the same, permanently.

Hungary

February

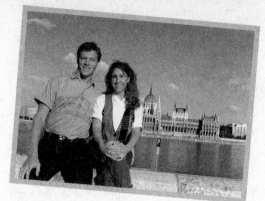

Youth

I met John Wendel at Lake Lytal Pool in suburban West Palm Beach. I was a lifeguard, just graduated from UNC. John was a high school teacher, swim coach, and former collegiate swimmer who practiced there.

I was transfixed watching him swim, his long, fluid strokes torpedoing his gorgeous body—he was a six-foot-one bronze statue—through the water.

John was so handsome that after two years of razzin' each other, I had a friend call and tell him he'd been selected for the Palm Beach Lifeguard Swimsuit Calendar.

John called me that night, the sap. I was in graduate school by then, and we were dating long-distance. "Hey, Susan, guess what?" he said. "I'm going to be in a swimsuit calendar. They let me pick the month. I asked for December because of your birthday."

"John . . ."

"Yes?"

"What day is it today?"

"Tuesday."

"No, what date?"

"April first . . ."

April Fools' Day. He laughed.

The April Fools' Day calendar-hunk caper started a tradition that continued all the way through Marina and Aubrey's chocolate-radish/slippery toilet classic. In twenty-three years, we have pulled some zingers, especially in the early days.

One year, I hid John's pricey bike, making him think it had been stolen.

"Goddammit!" he hollered as he hurtled his bike helmet across the apartment in frustration.

"April Fools!" I said.

The next year, oh boy, he got me back good. We were fooling around—I mean a moaner of a roll in the darkness—and John called out a name. "Beth! Beth!"

His old girlfriend.

'Twas I who went hurtling across the room that time.

I've always enjoyed that about John: he can laugh at himself. And he can laugh at me. Inside that beautiful body, I recognized a soul: a modest (yes, really), smart, steady-yet-fun soul.

When John talks about meeting me, though, he mentions my shorts. "She was wearing a University of North Carolina sweatshirt, and these blue shorts." He always stops there and shakes his head, thinking about my rear end.

I trust John with my life, and now with the lives of our children. In more than twenty years together, I have never seen him make a rash, senseless decision. (Except once, purchasing a used Ford with 80,000 miles on it.)

Even marriage was a practical decision. John received a Fulbright Commission berth to teach at a high school in Budapest, Hungary, in 1992. I had urged him to apply. Actually, I filled out the Fulbright application for him. He's an awful procrastinator.

John asked if I would go with him. We had to be married for me to accompany him on Fulbright functions, so one of us said, "Why don't we get hitched?"

We don't remember who.

And the other said, "Okay."

We casually mentioned it to my mother at Thanksgiving. Within days, she had the church, the pastor, the music, the organist. It was so swift, people musta wondered if I was pregnant. Let 'em wonder! I thought.

All I had to do was buy a wedding dress and show up. Which I did. Smiling the whole time. It was a small wedding, just family and our closest friends, at a nondenominational church.

Nancy, of course, was there.

We spent our wedding night at the local Hilton. Sat back in bed, looked at each other, and said, "What the hell did we just do?"

Five months later, we were living in Budapest.

People who know me a little think that doesn't sound like me at all. I'm a very together person. I don't make rash decisions.

When they know me better, they say, "That's so Susan." When I know what I want, I grab it. No waiting. No what-ifs. Just stop talking and do it already.

I wanted John, and I wanted Budapest. I was twenty-five.

I was an international studies major with a master's degree in my cherry-picked portable profession, journalism.

It was time for travel and adventure.

Budapest turned out to be one of the best decisions of our lives.

It was 1992, so the Berlin Wall had just come down. The city was rejoicing. Businesses going up. Statues coming down. It was the Wild West. Anything possible. A magnet for hucksters, youngsters, dead-enders, dreamers, anyone who wanted a chance.

And writers. I must have met a hundred. I met a recent Princeton graduate who was starting an English-language newspaper, the *Budapest Post*. Within a week, I was writing articles. Within two months, I was a senior editor, mentoring recent college journalism grads out to see the world.

At a news conference, I asked a question of Queen Elizabeth. At another, Boris Yeltsin. I flew on a relief mission over Bosnia and covered the Bulgarian rose harvest.

When I sat in the Hungarian Parliament, I'd see legislators with our paper, reading my articles. I was a twenty-five-year-old who didn't speak Hungarian, who had a translator for most of her interviews, and I was helping shape the opinions of legislators!

Then the kid ran out of money. The paper went belly-up. But someone knew someone at *Forbes*, the magazine of the ultra-wealthy. The paper was reborn as the *Budapest Sun*. My salary was now a pile of Hungarian cash. No checks or bank accounts. John and I hid the wad in a book in our apartment.

When we had money, we scoured the city, toured the nation and neighboring ones (we were almost killed in traffic in Turkey!), attended operas and concerts. We drank home-made wine in the midafternoon Budapest winter gloom.

When our cash ran out, we sat tight until the next payday. Laughing, talking, exploring each other. Surviving, like the newspaper, hand-to-mouth and day-to-day.

Those days, those adventures together, bonded us. Like glue on a piece of furniture, they were the invisible under-pinning that held us together for a lifetime, strained or un-strained.

The Fulbright ended. We came home, after two years abroad, to boring jobs and American excess. John didn't like his teaching position. I didn't like being a grunt at the *Palm Beach Post* after two years as a managing editor in Budapest. Even our small apartment with the air conditioner unit stuck in the dining-room window felt hollow.

And quick as a Florida thunderstorm, depression was upon me. *Thwack! Boom!*

I did not realize I was mentally ill until I'd lost fifteen pounds. Until my mind was so frazzled by lack of sleep, I'd have a panic attack when I lay down to try again.

In Hungary, every sense had been massaged with new sights, sounds, tastes, smells. Even the ordinary journalism assignments were fascinating.

Like when I was dispatched to cover the Eastern Euro-pean debut of the Chippendales, an America-based franchise of muscular men who stripped down to thong undies and thrusted for the hundreds of young women assembled.

"DO YA WANNA GET NASTY?" the buff boys hol-lered to the audience.

Which responded with absolute silence.

Delight.

Now I felt lousy, and everything seemed blah. John, increasingly depressed himself, felt powerless. We argued. I stayed with my sister for a brief spell. Stephanie drove me straight to the psychiatrist.

"Is the television talking to you?" the psychiatrist asked.

"I'm depressed, not psychotic!" I replied. The doc put me on an antidepressant. I felt much, much better.

I deeply believe we are the masters of our minds. That healthy, we can choose how we feel. But we are also our minds' lone caretakers, and we must keep them healthy. Now I practice my slow breathing, getting my Zen on. Living with joy.

Back then, John and I sought another post abroad, trying to recapture the wonder.

About a year later, we went to an international job fair for teachers. "There's a teaching position at a high school in Colombia," John pointed out. "They don't have spouse benefits . . . but they do have a job running the school yearbook."

My heart skipped. It was 1995, and Colombia was in the middle of a drug war. The year before, a soccer player on the national team had accidentally kicked the ball into his own goal during the World Cup. When he returned home, he was murdered. At that time, Colombia was widely considered the kidnapping capital of the world.

I agreed anyway. Life's an adventure, right? We signed a two-year contract.

This adventure wasn't so carefree. The cocaine wars were in their dying stages, but violence was rampant. Every corner shop had an armed guard. I'm talking ice cream shops, not banks. The school where John and I taught had a metal gate and armed guard turrets. There were men milling outside the gates with Italian suits, bad dental work, and machine guns. They were the students' bodyguards.

Kidnapping had devolved to a street-level crime: people were getting snatched on their way to the grocery store.

"I want to go home," I told John after seven months.

Honorable John didn't want to break our two-year contract. But I finally convinced him. We would leave at the end of the school year.

A month later, we hiked into the mountains during spring break. We were headed to La Ciudad Perdida (the Lost City), site of an ancient civilization hidden in the jungle for hundreds of years. It had only been rediscovered in the 1970s.

The hike was majestic. Mountains. Canopied forest. Streams. Toucans flying across terraced landings.

It was also long days of walking uphill. With a guide and armed bodyguards, because this was guerrilla country. No showers. No toilets. Our group slept in hammocks on the second story of open-sided huts. On the first story, a fire was kept lit to ward off the bugs. The smoke kept me awake.

By the sixth day, I couldn't take it anymore. It was raining. I was sick. I snapped. "That's it," I said, on the verge of tears. "I'm tired. I'm hungry. I'm filthy and nauseous and sore. And I think I'm pregnant!"

I turned to stomp off into the jungle and slammed right into a support post for the hut. I fell flat on my back in the mud. *Splat.*

And that's how John found out about our first child. Then did the math—back to our celebration on the night we'd decided to go home.

Life is perfect like that. Otherwise I would have delayed and delayed having children, wanting to travel more. I was thirty years old.

The pregnancy began as twins and was high-risk. We couldn't afford health insurance without our jobs, so we had to stay in Colombia for another year. Talk about nerve-racking— try being pregnant at an altitude of 9,000 feet in the kidnapping capital of the world.

I miscarried one twin.

Then, a week short of due, the remaining baby stopped moving. I was at school, working, so I talked to the nurse.

"Eat sugar," she said.

It didn't work. The baby didn't start moving again. By the afternoon, we were in panic mode. John ran out into the rain to hail a cab to the hospital, couldn't find one, and stopped the next best thing.

"Come on," he said, dripping wet. "I got us a ride."

It was the kindergarten school bus. Full of children. Sure enough, it went right past the hospital, opened its hydraulic doors with a sigh, and dropped us off.

"What have you had to eat in the last six hours?" the anesthesiologist asked.

I had taken the nurse's sugar advice. "Two Cokes and three brownies," I replied.

The doc gave me that look. You know the one. Pathetic.

An hour later, I was in the operating room. The baby was breech, and the cord was wrapped around its neck. It would have to be a C-section. John watched them make the incision. Then his face turned gray and he started to sway.

"Unlock your knees!" I yelled. "Don't pass out!"

He did and stayed upright. I heard a cry and asked him the baby's sex.

"I think it's a girl."

"What do you mean, 'you think?' "

"Well, everything's kinda swollen."

We could not name our child without meeting her. So a few hours later, in a hospital bed, I asked John what name popped into his head when he saw our little girl.

"Brie," he said.

Like all babies, she had been covered with white goo.

I rolled my eyes and decided on Ella.

The notary said the name would not be approved. In Spanish, *ella* means "she." Nope, it wouldn't do. The woman didn't care if it was common in English.

So we gazed at our baby for days. At the wonder of her. Finally, we named her Marina.

Partly because it sounded Spanish. Partly because it was Greek, like my mother. Mostly because she had blue eyes. A calm, gentle blue that reminded me of the ocean on a sunny day, a place I always felt safe and warm.

Oh, Marina. Beautiful girl. I remember holding you. And learning to nurse you.

My milk came in full force the night we arrived home from the hospital. "You look like an exotic dancer," John said of my supersized self. This was the same man who had brought my thong underwear and skinny jeans to the hospital, as if I was going to immediately spring back into my old shape.

"Please find me a breast pump!" I begged. "And not a cheap one. The Cadillac of breast pumps." It felt like my breasts were going to explode.

But oh, the amusement of thinking of all that now. I've relived with joy those nights of pain, when my tiny child bit me like a demon. That sweet life in my arms. That milky breath. My husband at my side, bringing her to me to nurse in the moonlight. Then laying our baby back so gently in her bassinet.

Marina, you put an end to our traveling days.

Marina, you catapulted us into the parent years. That phase of life where days are interminable and years are over in an instant.

A time I wish was longer. A time I would not trade for anything.

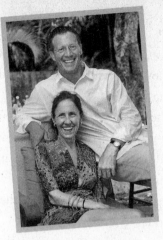

A Couple

We tried for another child awhile before he came—a son, Aubrey, in 2001. Such a content, adorable baby—he was as chubby and content as a Buddha—that we mulled over another, and *shazam!* there he came, Wesley, in 2003.

Suddenly, I had three children under the age of six, while working full-time. Naturally, our marriage suffered. John and I became like furniture to one another.

We were so strained, we considered separation.

But as with an old comfy chair, we were reluctant to let it go.

Both sets of our parents have been married fifty years. We thought of their example. We stuck it out, moment by moment.

We rarely did anything alone, just the two of us. John had quit teaching. Why? Try forty students, twenty-five desks, and twenty books. He became a pharmaceutical sales rep for

GlaxoSmithKline. Occasionally, he would win a Glaxo trip. We went to Vancouver in 2006. For a decade, that was our one big couple trip.

Then, in the summer of 2009, John won a trip to Hawaii. It was during the packing and planning that I noticed my withered hand. I delayed a follow-up neurologist visit till after the trip because, let me tell you, when you're looking at an all-expenses-paid vacation to Hawaii, there is not a whit wrong in the world.

Forget temporary health setbacks. That summer, my chief concern was finding (tasteful) silver heels to match my (tasteful) silver bangles to match my favorite blue tube dress for the luau.

And did my turquoise batik sarong truly match my swimsuit? Oh my! Now that's a reason to worry.

In August, John and I left the kids with Nancy and Stephanie and flew to a Technicolor dream. The Royal Hawaiian Hotel in Honolulu was resplendent with antiques and painted an elegant pink, unlike the cotton-candy schmaltz of south Florida. The Pacific Ocean was violet offshore, aqua inland. The leis glowed magenta, and the evening sky orange.

Glaxo had the whole trip planned, an activity for every minute. A pig roast luau. A dance. John and I took a surfing lesson and rode horses at a ranch overlooking the ocean. We stood on a cliff, side by side, and watched a huge mango sun sink into the sea.

A moment to remember, like John as he glided through the swimming pool in 1991. Or ice in the Danube during our first year in Budapest.

Near the end, we kayaked with a guide to Lanikai Beach, oft-voted one of the most beautiful beaches in the world. The sand was white with the texture of flour, but no powdery residue. I called it "magic sand."

Just offshore was a coral reef, with stands rising out of the water as the tide receded. We swam on it, watching tropical fish and anemones wave to us in the current. The colors glowed: orange, yellow, purple, blue.

The peace was shattered by a pharma rep from New York, panicked over a pair of nurse sharks. He climbed atop the reef, hollering, "Shawk! Shawk!" It might have been funny if he had not damaged a thousand generations of coral.

Dolt, I thought, plunging my head into the wondrous clear water, sharks and all.

There were moments of concern in Hawaii—when I couldn't tug my tube dress down or manage a skewer of shrimp with my weak left hand—but I hardly thought of that. Back in West Palm Beach, I made an appointment to see the neurologist, then stared at a photo of myself on Lanikai Beach.

The perfect screen saver. The last healthy moment of my life.

I told John he didn't need to come with me to see Dr. Zuniga, the neurologist. He insisted on coming anyway.

"Why?" I asked.

He did not tell me at the time, but he had been discussing my symptoms with his doctor friends. He was so concerned, he had begun pulling over on the side of the road between sales calls, too worried to drive.

John was quiet while Dr. Zuniga examined me, tested my muscles, then scratched his head and said he was puzzled.

"So you don't think she has ALS?" John blurted out.

"Oh, no," Dr. Zuniga said quickly. "Susan's so young. And it's contained in the hand. ALS usually spreads quickly."

John fell back in his chair. "Thank God," he said. "Thank God."

I looked at John. Then Dr. Zuniga. "What's ALS?" I asked.

John wouldn't discuss it. I Googled it. Once.

It rattled me so, I never did it again.

Instead, I went into denial. John never did. After twenty years, he was more attuned to me than any person on the planet. He noticed a slight slur in my speech in late 2009, long before anyone else. He said not a word to me about it for six months.

It was even longer before he admitted that he would roll over in the middle of the night to put his arm around me, and that he could feel, because he knew my topography so well, that something was wrong.

When I was pregnant, he would wrap his arms around my expanding body. He loved to feel the changes.

Now he felt me wasting away.

He was afraid. But he did not pull away. Moment by moment, and muscle lost by muscle lost, John and I grew together. Through all the bright-line moments, he was supportive and steady.

Steady as a trapeze artist. Even as reality became grimmer and grimmer, as the thin wire rose higher and higher, and there was farther to fall.

By September 2011, I was wound tight. My appetite had been diminished for months, part of my ALS. It all but disappeared as I watched Mom starving in the hospital, her digestive system so beaten she couldn't ingest anything by mouth.

It was a celebration when she was allowed an ice chip.

I was so tense, I ground my jaw to the point of pain. I couldn't sleep. I would go an entire day without eating and not even be tummy-rumbly at the end. I dropped two sizes, to 00 pants.

Our friends tried to help, each in their own way.

Which, for one, meant gifting us with a large bag of marijuana.

This friend had long battled addictions of all kinds. He told me my situation had inspired him to live clean. Instead of throwing out his pot—"Impossible! It's really good shit!" he said—he was donating it to me. "You have much more use for it than I do, Susan. It will help with your pain."

I could count on one hand the number of times I had smoked pot in the preceding fifteen years. I had never bought it, and only inhaled on the rare occasion when it was offered (by my birth mama, for instance). I had a respectable job and three children. Those were my priorities, not reefer.

Plus, it was illegal.

But . . .

I was stressed over Mom to the point of wearing down my teeth. I was in pain from my broken clavicle, which had to set naturally. And I was terminally ill.

I needed a freakin' break.

Pot, I remembered from my college days, usually made

me eat and laugh like the dickens. Both of which I needed to do.

I enlisted John to the cause. After all the difficult tasks of the last two years—tasks more mental than physical, although the physical period was coming—this was a request he didn't mind.

Ideally, we would have smoked up at home, eaten an entire pint of Sea Salt Caramel gelato and watched the Science Channel stoned to the bejesus. But not with our children nearby.

So John and I plotted a night out to smoke pot and eat ourselves silly at our favorite Mexican restaurant.

Now we had another problem: where could two responsible adults smoke pot and not have to drive impaired to their Mexican chowdown?

The restaurant was in downtown West Palm Beach, near the courthouse where I had worked as a reporter. A courthouse where people arrested for marijuana-related crimes appear every day. We should, we both realized, park and smoke, then walk to the restaurant. And the closest site devoid of traffic and pedestrians was said courthouse.

So that night, we pulled up in our van on an empty street aside the ginormous dark courthouse. Crept up, really, like two criminals in a bad cop drama. John rolled a joint, and—doh!—a light went off in my head. Sheriff's deputies patrolled the building's perimeter. Not a good spot, ya dolt!

Thinking I was so clever, I told John to pull north a block to another dark, deserted street. Now we were beside a tall hedge and the offices of the prosecutors, including the chief prosecutor, who was no fan of my reporting.

He was a thin-skinned politician who resented it when reporters asked real questions like: "Precisely how many tax-payer dollars did you spend hiring a fashion consultant for your office?"

Perfect. We fired up.

Pretty soon, a haze built up in the van. I put my window down and puffed away, exhaling out the window. John and I laughed about how we looked like a Cheech and Chong skit, just two heads in the cloud.

Then we heard voices. They were coming from a few feet away, on the other side of the hedge.

Here's how Cannabisconsumer.org describes the effect of pot: "Cannabis use can increase focus and concentration, making a person's moods, sensations, and experience seem more intense. Your heart might feel like it's pounding, the music fantastic, this is the best dessert you've ever eaten and wow, get a load of how beautiful nature is."

And then, FAR DOWN the page, another effect: paranoia.

Yes, pot makes you intently focused. How yummy those Cheetos are, how cool those space wormholes. But God help you if your thoughts turn paranoid, because those are amplified, too.

Those voices in the hedge—and let me tell you, they were enhanced to seem like they were coming from right inside the van—sent one thought rattling around in my head: Pot is illegal. What we are doing is illegal.

And like fools we had brought the whole flippin' bag of weed. Which surely ramped up our chance of being arrested if caught, right?

I told John to drive away from the voices. No, not so fast.

Okay, too slow. He eased up the block and I turned, real casual, to look behind the hedge.

And there they were: two sheriff's deputies, leaning against their squad cars, talking. I had been blowing pot smoke *toward* the cops, from six feet away.

Suddenly I was very stoned. And very paranoid.

Surely they musta smelled it.

Surely they were comin' after us.

Surely there would be a manhunt for our van, and they'd run my tag and know it was me.

And surely my ass would land in the newspaper—"*Post* Crime Reporter Arrested: Top Prosecutor Thrilled!"

I wanted to go home. But John's stoned mind was intently focused on something else: Nachos.

Again, the man can eat at any time.

We walked to the Mexican restaurant, arm in arm. I could hardly eat. I was so nervous, I scanned the crowd for deputies coming for me with handcuffs unlocked. Everyone in the place was glancing our way. And the waitress kept smiling. Why? She knew. Everyone knew.

John finished his meal and mine. All that trouble, and I ate maybe four bites of Mexican food.

We left without incident and took a cab home.

As I lay down that night, I realized I was still stoned. I vowed never to do such a foolish thing again.

"Next time we're staying home," I told John. "Eatin' gelato and watching the Science Channel."

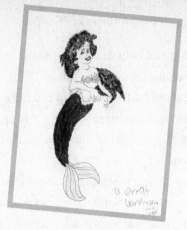

The Conversation

It wasn't until Christmas, when I'd finally had the chance to experience some peace within my illness, that I became concerned for John. He was strong, but he internalized. He rarely, if ever, talked of how he felt.

I heard him say: "I'm glad I'm a pharmaceutical rep, because between appointments, I can pull over to the side of the road and cry."

I worried because he was the one Aubrey went to and asked, "Does Mom have muscular dystrophy?"

"No," John told him. "But what she has is similar."

When I think of which role is worse—to be the spouse dying or the spouse surviving—I think it's the latter. The survivor will experience the same grief, will live the grief of the children, then must assume the responsibilities and slog on.

Already, I knew, the responsibilities were overwhelming John. The cooking. The cleaning. Trying to get our children to stop bickering and help. It was like an alarm clock went off every fifteen minutes with those three.

John dressed and bathed me. Paid the bills. Prepared food. Fed me when I was too tired to hold a fork, talked for me when my tired tongue slurred words so badly no one but him could understand.

He remembered appointments. Attended school meetings. Kept our family calendar. He took over from me as the family organizer and information center, the parent who always knew what was going on.

He was the one who had to dress his fashion-conscious wife. The buttons, zippers, snaps, hooks, ties, sashes, belts, pads, buckles, the underwear that can only be worn with certain items of clothes.

"I can't wear those," I told John one day, when he brought me a pair of cotton underwear. "I need a slippery pair."

"What does that mean?"

"A pair that won't stick to the dress."

"Huh?"

"You know when you see a woman's backside, and her dress is plastered to her butt like a piece of chewing gum? That's because she doesn't have slippery underwear."

He sighed. "I need a manual."

I knew John was hurting, but he didn't want to take an antidepressant. He had a friend he could talk to, he told me, a woman who had lost her husband in a bicycle accident. They talked of which was better: a sudden absence or inevitable decline.

I urged him to go to the doctor. He had always been so calm and reasonable. Now he was yelling at the children and tearing up at stoplights.

Aubrey came to me one day. "He yelled at me to practice my trumpet. He told Wesley to go draw pictures. Mom, Wesley draws pictures all day. That's all he does."

It's true—because of his Asperger's, Wesley often draws for hours. He has an extraordinary ability to reproduce things he sees, especially princesses and his beloved Piglet.

"I know, honey," I told Aubrey, hugging him as best I could. "Please practice your trumpet."

John finally realized he needed help one day as he dressed me. Each tie, each lace, each zipper, he wept.

John's boss was a Jamaican fellow whom he admired, a man with a peace about him. "Sometimes ya just need a bump, mon," he told John.

John started the antidepressant Wellbutrin. He cried less, yelled less, chuckled more at the TV commercials.

He still had his doubts. Not about the unmanliness of taking mood medicine—John's not macho—but about its effects.

"It keeps you in a box," he said. "It cuts off the highs and the lows." He didn't like not being able to feel the same joy, but he knew it was necessary. "The lows are just so hard," he said. "So hard. And they are with me all the time."

I helped him as best I could. I tried to keep drama, complaints, requests for help, and tears to a minimum. I refrained from declaring things like, "Honey, I can no longer lift my left arm," because what an unending cascade of "I'm sorrys" that would start.

I had a uterine ablation, a surgical procedure that scraped away the lining of the uterus, reducing blood flow. I didn't want John to have to deal with periods, too.

We hired a woman to clean and help around the house, a Haitian woman named Yvette. Nancy recommended her. We all love her.

Yet I still wanted John to help me, feed me, bathe me. No one made me feel safer than he did. He knew just how to lift me gently and support me as I walked.

We talked about everything. I may have been circumspect with others, but with John no subject was off limits.

It was hard for me to say, "When I can no longer stand . . . ," "When I can no longer eat . . . ," "When I can no longer speak . . ."

It was hard for John to hear.

Hard. But necessary.

I made clear my end-of-life wishes and my hopes for him when I die: that he remarry. That he find some gorgeous woman who (unlike *moi*) would do triathlons with him. That he bring her to live in our home, no guilt.

It didn't even need to be said, "Choose someone whom our children also adore," such is my absolute faith in his judgment.

John listened when I spoke of the future, but rarely replied. He focused on immediate tasks. He almost never spoke of his own hopes in a life without me.

Until late one night, after a few drinks, he got serious and said he was ashamed to tell me something.

Lord, I thought, what could it be?

He said that after I die, he wanted to go back to school to become a physician's assistant. That it was a better career for a single father of three, and that he believed he would be good at it and enjoy it.

I was thrilled! A new career, a giant change-up in his life, would speed burial of the past.

"Don't ever feel guilty to tell me what you hope for without me," I said, my curled fingers resting on his hand. "It comforts me, John. It makes me happy."

I now study anatomy. I had often struggled to explain to John precisely where the itch was I needed him to scratch. So I am learning the lingo: "Right posterior second metacarpal, please."

He scratches in the exact right place. I smile. John is learning anatomy too. He is learning to be a physician's assistant with a real patient.

I am doing what I can to launch him into a life without me.

Joyfully.

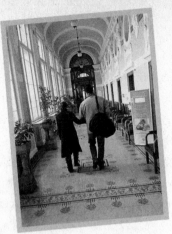

Budapest

Our special place was Budapest. When John and I talked about the past, as we often did, our thoughts always came back to this city where we spent our first two years of marriage. The place where we laid the foundation for our lives together.

After the wonder of the Yukon with Nancy, Budapest was the place I thought of first. It was our twentieth wedding anniversary that year. I wanted to spend it with John in the place where our married life began.

Whatever the future, John and I told ourselves, we have today. We have old memories to rekindle and new memories to make.

The Hungarian cold hit us hard. John and I were used to south Florida winters and had forgotten how chilling Budapest in February could be. I was a tropical girl. Why, I wondered, was I always traveling into the cold?

Then we heard the warm laugh, booming across the airport. A memory from two decades before.

"*Szervuszstok!*" our old friend Feri Der shouted, greeting us in Hungarian with hugs and kisses. John had met Feri during our first stay. They played on a baseball team together, a Hungarian passion at the time (though John was only one on the team who knew all the rules). I had not seen Feri in Hungary for twenty years, and there he was.

"*Szervuszstok*, my friends. *Szervuszstok!* So good to see you. I'll get the car."

When we left Budapest in 1994, Russian and East German autos had chugged along its streets. One, the Trabant, powered by a mix of oil and gas, spewed so much pollution that building facades crumbled. Feri drove a truck called a Barkas, a classic piece of East German technology that always broke down.

This time, as John helped me to the curb, we noticed a white Cadillac Escalade. "Man, that's odd to see here," John said.

And out of the Caddy hopped Feri, laughing.

On the ride from the airport, we saw the effect of twenty years. Gas stations, German groceries, billboards, giant box stores, and—Lord help me—strip malls. Once-dark streets awash in neon. Renaissance buildings with shiny new drugstores on their first floors.

Don't miss the old, I told myself. Embrace the new.

In 1994, Feri had been living in a shanty in a Budapest suburb, building his dream home. The shanty was little more than a plywood box with a cot. Feri scraped together money bill by bill. John had helped him build clay walls nearly two feet thick with a trowel and shovel, one foot at a time. One day, they went together to the forest and selected the home's master beam.

Now we pulled up to the completed dream: a square, two-story traditional farmhouse in the middle of Budapest. A piece of the past in a post-Soviet world.

Feri showed us each detail: the scalloped roof tiles, heated floors, custom bread oven, a woven-branch fence that offered a relief from the chain fences that fronted the other yards. Feri had wrought the iron window latches himself. "A hundred and twenty-four of them!"

And his sweetest spot—a large underground wine cellar. The walls were made of special stones brought from Hungary's winemaking region. On them grew a black mold that imparts taste to the wine.

In that cellar, Feri made magic—red, white, sweet, dry, and a Hungarian firewater called *pálinka*. In no time, we were taste-testing.

"Relieve your glasses of their air!" he shouted. "It's so good you're here. It's like you never left."

All of Hungary was around us. All our memories. The opera. The historic buildings. The Parliament. The countryside. Yet there was no place I'd rather be than the wine cellar with my husband and our best Hungarian friend.

The occasion called for a special Hungarian stew, Feri said. Traditional, cooked over an open fire. "Tomorrow we slaughter the rabbits. John, you will do so as well."

"You going to do it?" I asked the next morning in Feri's guest room, as John buttoned me into my coat.

John is a gentle soul—never hunted, never handled a gun nor wanted to, and certainly never bashed in a rabbit's head, strung it up by its hind legs, and slit its throat.

"I guess," he said with a deep sigh.

John helped me into my long black coat, my boots and brace, and parked me outside on the porch so I could watch.

After some *pálinka* shots, Feri selected the first rabbit to die, a twelve-pound gray-and-white, the largest of his collection.

He bashed it to break its neck, strung it up, and sliced.

"You now," he said to John.

Together they killed three rabbits, skinned and gutted them, chopped them in pieces, John grimacing most the time.

As I watched, I thought more of John than of the kill, of how bizarre it was to see him doing something I had never seen him do before. And how comforting the sense it gave—that he will have another life one day, without me, full of new adventures.

Feri's partner, Vikki, brought fixings for the stew: a mound of chopped onion, tubes of spicy paprika cream, a block of lard.

She made dumplings by hand. Feri boiled the rabbits in a cauldron over the fire, adding wine and water and the fixings.

He brought one of his finest wines from the cellar, a cabernet, liquid velvet. We huddled round the fire, our glasses propped in the snow.

I am so glad to be here, I thought. I am so glad to be alive.

Feri spent several days with us, laughing, breaking into show tunes, playing his accordion. He took us to public medicinal baths, drove us around his city, helped suit me up in winter gear. He was a constant presence who lifted our spirits—and occasionally my body, too.

He stuffed us—with wild boar, a smorgasbord of *kolbász*

from venison and other animals, and sour cherry dumplings he fell in love with while working in Russia.

"Eat, eat," he would say. "There is always more."

Feri had been an executive with Avon, soaring to success on ingenuity and pluck. As their general manager in Russia, he raised sales by $100 million.

"The Russian women, they must eat lipstick for breakfast," he said, grinning.

Feri told John and me of a seemingly intractable personal problem he was having.

"Well, if you can't change the situation, change your attitude," I told him. "You are the master of your mind."

"That's so American," Feri said, rolling his eyes.

But he kissed and hugged me all the same.

It snowed hard. That was another difference in Budapest this time around, the big, wet snow. John and I had been in Budapest snows before. But we had never seen her gray, gray streets frosted pure white.

We wanted to be out in the enchantment, even though walking in snow was like walking through cookie dough for me.

No bother. You only live once.

John suited me up: coat, brace, boots. This was another good thing about living in Florida, we realized. Warm-weather clothes are easier than cold, especially when you cannot use your hands.

I've kissed cold weather good-bye forever now.

But that day it was magnificent. White. New. Barely touched.

We set out in the city to hunt for a restaurant we had

eaten at many times. We couldn't remember its name, only its enormous portions of goose and sweet cabbage with apples worth traipsing through anything to eat again.

And I remembered the location, on a small avenue off a large central square called Deák Ferenc Tér—a place I passed daily when we lived here.

We traipsed and traipsed, around icy spots on the sidewalks, down cobblestone streets, trying not to slip, trip, or otherwise fall. I grew tired. Could barely lift my feet. John wiped snow off a bench and left me there to scamper ahead and scout the scene.

But no matter how we approached Deák Tér, we could not get our bearings. We could not find the little avenue. The billboards on the square and new shops made it unrecognizable to me.

We abandoned the search, saying, "Ah, well, probably closed anyhow."

After all, the newspaper I'd helped start, the *Budapest Sun*, had folded three years before.

One day we met up with a former colleague from the *Sun*, Steve Saracco. We asked about the restaurant. He pointed it out, exactly where it had always been, as he walked with us to the subway at Deák Tér.

John and Steve helped me down the stairs to the subway entrance. It smelled just as it had twenty years ago, of fried dough and fuel. We bought the same little flimsy ticket, punched it in the same little machine, boarded the same grimy escalator cycling too fast. We waited on the same platform, underneath the same hideous orange ceiling for the same blue train.

Sadness hijacked my spirit. We bid good-bye to Steve, and I wept uncontrollably.

"Why are you crying?" John asked.

"I can't even find words to explain."

On our wedding anniversary—Valentine's Day—John and I set out alone. A special night, arranged by Feri, in a suite at the Hotel Gellert.

The art nouveau Gellert, completed in 1918, was like a beautiful grandmother. Worn, outdated, but with classic style. Its stained glass and wrought-iron accents were a delight, even overlaid with Soviet-era eyesores, fluorescent lighting, and bulbous sign lettering from the 1970s.

Feri had snagged us the Richard Nixon suite, so named after the president who laid his head there twice.

"I know. I know. No Tricky Dick jokes," John said to me.

The room's small balcony overlooked the Danube River, ice floes drifting upon it.

We donned the bathrobes provided, and John carried me down the stairs to the spa. We parted into the steamy, sex-segregated indoor baths.

I sat alone in the 100-degree water, nestled as close to the font of the thermal mineral spring as possible. Above me were blue-and-green mosaic-tiled domes. Honeyed light streamed through glass ceiling tiles into the steamy, cavernous room.

I studied the women—young and old, bulbous and sinewy, naked and suited. I studied how they glided across the wet tile floors, how they descended the steps into the water so gracefully, how the light glistened upon their muscled limbs.

And I wondered how the hell I was going to get out.

My trips weakened me. I realized that even before Wreck Beach. They broke down muscles that would never grow back.

But they strengthened my mind. My heart.

A fair trade?

By Budapest, I was limping badly. Every time I lifted my left foot to step, the front of it dropped, causing me to trip on my own toes.

I wore a brace, which helped prevent that. But there in the women's-only bath, I had no brace.

And no husband to lean on.

I sat back in the pool. I had time. This, after all, was the Budapest I loved. The city sits on a vast network of hot mineral springs and is renowned in Europe for its medicinal baths. Baths centuries old, saunas and thermal pools, salt rooms and steam rooms designed to cure any number of ills. Baths are such an integral part of health care that some offer dental services on-site.

I thought of that day in Canada's Yukon Territory with Nancy, and our magical dip in the outdoor hot spring. There, for a moment, I saw myself old.

Here, I felt myself young.

I exited the pool, clutching the brass handrails at the stairs. Stepped onto the wet tile in the honey-lit center of the room. The ladies in the pools stared as I struggled in the spotlight on the slippery stage—focusing my cosmic zoom on each step, trying not to eat the tile floor.

This is one of those moments I have to choose, I told myself. To feel sorry for myself or not.

I chose the latter.

"How'd ya do?" John asked when we met up again.

"Fine," I said, excising any drama.

Upstairs in our Tricky Dick suite, we bathed, our first moments completely alone and at peace in a long time.

As he shampooed my hair, I asked John if he was okay with our decisions thus far—not to go Google crazy and hunt false ALS cures, not to clamor to be part of a clinical trial only to receive a placebo, not to falsely hope a drug would come.

Our decision to just be. Accept. Live with joy. And die with joy, too.

"I don't know how you do it," John said. "If I were you, I would probably drive myself into a tree."

"I have thought of that," I said.

"Please don't."

"I won't. Because the children would never understand."

"Good."

"Absent that, I would free you of this burden."

"It is not a burden," John said. "The least I can do for you is everything."

He lifted me from the tub, dried me, combed out my snarled hair, fastened my bra. "This is the one I hook on the loosest notch, right?"

"You are getting good at this!" I smiled.

For the first time, John put stockings on me—silken black ones so sheer he could easily punch a thumb through. "Careful!" I said.

He slipped a sweater dress over my head, knelt, and directed my feet into my brace and boots. "Toe curled?"

My toes had no muscles. Putting on shoes could curl them under my foot, causing considerable pain when I walked.

"No."

Once again, John negotiated me into the long black coat, bum arm first. "Thumb bent backward!" I said. I didn't have the strength to push it through the sleeve myself.

And finally a black hat. "Flower not fully forward, please. Looks like I have a bunch of broccoli on my forehead."

On the way to dinner, I tripped and fell, tearing a hole in my stockings.

"Wanna go back to the room and change?" John said.

"No. I just want to eat and enjoy."

And there, in a quiet corner of the hotel restaurant, we did.

We feasted on five courses, each with its own wine, laughing at the English translations—"flap mushrooms"—looking back at the menu descriptions, tasting for every ingredient described.

The walnut polenta and ginger of the carrot soup.

The green mussel inside ravioli.

The *mangalica* pork, from a Hungarian pig with twice the flavor of regular pork.

The marzipan and raspberry gelatin of the dessert tray.

We savored each sip—red, white, pink, dry, sweet.

We talked of the things and people we had to be thankful for. We laughed at how on that same night twenty years ago, after we married, we both had said, "What the hell did we just do?"

We talked of how going abroad had catapulted us into life together and what good partners we had made.

The waiter asked if he could go ahead and bring the check, as the restaurant was closing.

We ended with a glass of fine champagne.

As we walked out, I leaned heavily on John, knowing there was no way I could make it back to the room on my own.

Finally there, he undressed me, piece by piece, and carried me to bed.

The Cruise

March

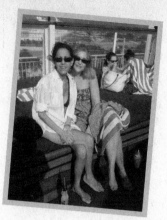

My Sister Steph

The cruise ship seesawed on the roiling ocean. Passengers tottered sideways, arms stretched to balance, stumbling to handrails.

I clung to my sister Steph like a koala on a tree.

It was less than three weeks since Hungary, a trip that both energized and tired me. At this point in my illness, I couldn't balance alone on terra firma. That ship, on that windy night, was like dancing on a hammock.

"What brain surgeon thought of a cruise?" Steph said.

"You, my dear."

Sweet Steph. I think she saw my other trips and decided, Uh-uh, not for me. Steph is a homebody who doesn't like to fly.

Yukon? No. Hungary? No way. Cyprus, the trip I was planning next? That was my special thing. Steph has promised to take my children there one day, and I believe she will, white-knuckled the whole flight. But that's for after I'm gone.

For now, Stephanie and I didn't have a special thing, at

least not travel-wise. We were close as kids, though rarely did our social lives intersect. And then, before ya know it, I was traveling the world, and she was married with two babies.

"I thought about what I was missing," Stephanie says of those days when John and I were traveling in Europe and South America. She was living less than a mile from Mom's house, raising two kids. "But that's not me. I'm a nurturer. I like being a mom. And I'm good at it."

She's right. Just ask her two fabulous boys, William and Stephen. Her second husband, Don, is the happiest man I know.

And her first husband, Bill, still adores her.

Ask my children. When I began struggling with walking after the Yukon, Aunt Stephanie started coming over every day after her job teaching respiratory therapy at a local college.

Sitting in the backyard, sipping some girlie drink. (But only sipping; Stephanie has the alcohol tolerance of a mosquito.) Watching my kids. Talking about Mom, which helped us love her more. That was our thing.

So for our journey together, Stephanie chose the simplest trip possible. She treated me to a cruise that left port a few miles from our home. It was our first trip together as adults.

I had no clue she had never been on a cruise.

"I envisioned umbrella drinks, sun, and smooth sailing," Steph said, trying to hold us both upright. "This is a freaking nightmare!"

It was so rough, we beelined for the dining room well before dinner to minimize walking. We sat in the low leather chairs of the bar. "Let's have a drink. A brandy," I said.

"Gosh no!" she said.

I looked over. Steph was sitting with her eyes closed, her chair bobbing with the sea.

"I'm just trying to go with it," Steph said. "I keep telling myself it's like a hammock. Try to go with the rolls."

"Do you get seasick?"

"I go green looking at boats."

We sat silently awhile. An entertainer took to the mike, singing, playing guitar, joking with the audience.

"I'll go to the room for our dinner reservation card," Steph said suddenly. And just as suddenly she staggered out, leaving me alone in the bar.

She didn't make it to the room. Her stomach bum-rushed her on the elevator. She had to pinch her lips together with her fingers to keep the rising tide down.

She made it out of the elevator, thank goodness. And ten steps away to an ashtray, where she erupted.

Some sympathetic soul handed a barf bag over her shoulder, avoiding the line of fire. Bag in hand, she stumbled down the hallway, the staff already heading toward the ashtray with vacuums and towels.

She heard a man upchucking and crying two cabins away. "Man up, will ya?" she muttered.

She crashed onto the bed and closed her eyes. Each time she opened them, she vomited.

She panicked at the thought of me stranded at the bar, knowing there was no way I could walk on my own, or even push myself out of the chair.

She crawled to the door. Opened it. Called out. Our steward, an Indonesian man named Budi, answered.

"Sister. Susan. Bar. Needs help," Stephanie said, pausing to quell the queasiness. "Can't walk. Black pants. Poncho."

"Poncho? What's a poncho?" a bewildered Budi said.

"Like a cape. Superman."

Budi looked more bewildered.

"Ponytail. Go!"

She sent Budi with my dinner card and an antinausea pill.

By this time, I knew she was sick. For fifteen minutes, I had struggled to rise on my own from the low chair, stumbling back time and again.

"Cut her off!" hollered the entertainer.

Good thing I can't lift my middle fingers, I thought, else that entertainer would be getting a two-fisted bird. I had not had a drop to drink.

But the music was so loud, I couldn't project my voice enough to ask for help. I slumped back, accepting my fate. What will be, will be.

Eventually, an Asian ship employee approached and handed me a pill. Budi.

Budi gestured as if vomiting. I understood. Stephanie was down for the count.

This is gonna be interesting, I thought.

I placed Budi's hand on my shoulder, to signal I needed help standing. He fumbled with how to hold me, nearly knocking me over when he placed his hand across my lower back and pushed forward.

"Just get a wheelchair!" called out another employee.

At the cabin, Steph answered the door, hunched over, a green ghost. "Thank goodness you're here," she said.

We both lay on the bottom bunk, neither able to climb the ladder to the top. Steph's legs quivered as she lay, eyes closed, trying not to vomit again.

"There is water here. Drink some," I said.

"I can't keep it down. Want me to take your shoes and braces off?"

"No," I said. "Just rest."

We lay with our eyes closed, rocked back and forth by the ocean, listening to the waves crashing aside the ship, and fell asleep.

The next morning, we awoke to stillness—the ship had docked in Freeport, the Bahamas, a mere sixty-eight miles from home in West Palm Beach.

We stayed onboard the near-empty vessel, lingering over breakfast on white linen, the table overlooking an electric blue bay.

Steph was back to normal. She looked beautiful in the soft sunlight, the hazel of her large eyes glowing.

I was so happy with the tiny coffee cups I could easily hold. Each time the waiter poured more, Steph opened the cream and sugar for me. Oh, life's little pleasures.

She brought me waffles and eggs and fruit from the self-serve buffet. I eat at a glacial pace, the muscles of my mouth failing. Patiently, Steph waited.

The waiters finally asked us to leave. They had to prepare the table for lunch.

We changed into bathing suits and lounged around the ship. Under canopies on deck. At the pool.

We talked and talked, which is something Steph and I have rarely done before, just the two of us. No cell phones.

No kids (five between us). No pets (six). No friends (hundreds). No distractions.

We cried together. Really cried.

The conversation turned to my birth mother.

Over the last couple years, as I have peeled back the layers of my own heritage, Steph has expressed nothing but support and happiness for me. And a few times, in the most tenuous way, she has said *maybe* she would look for her own birth mother.

"I so wish she would look for me," Steph said, which broke my heart.

Now here is where you have to understand Steph's personality. You see, Steph is a hard-core addict. Her juice? Her buzz? The thing that gives her a glorious high, leaving her glowing inside?

Pleasing people.

All her life, Steph has made pleasing others more important than satisfying herself. I remember one Thanksgiving at her house, she invited a female friend who does little but annoy her and poke fun at her.

I am protective of my big sis. I could see how much the woman's nagging was hurting Steph. So I basically threw her out.

"Why the hell did you invite her?" I asked.

"Because I was afraid she might get upset if I didn't," Steph said.

To which I am certain I gave a major eye roll.

The next Thanksgiving, Steph got a hair bolder and did not invite her friend. Rather, she asked all us family members not to drive our cars to her house so no one would know she was having a gathering and be hurt they weren't invited.

Mind you, it was Thanks-effing-giving.

In our family, we are conditioned not to talk candidly of our most trenchant emotions. Or hurts. Or fears. But that day on the ship, Steph told me one of her fears: that even mentioning her birth mother would hurt Mom and Dad.

She worried the search would be disappointing. Would she even like the lady? Would the lady even want to meet her?

The only thing Steph knows is that the woman was seventeen years old when she gave birth at Good Samaritan Medical Center in December 1964.

"A baaaaby!" Steph said with empathy.

I wanted to drop the emotional hammer on Steph and tell her my thought: that I would very much like for her to try to find her birth mother before I die, so that I might meet her and say, "You brought to life an exceptional human being who God divined my sister. And it was indeed divine. Thank you."

But on the ship, in a rare moment of self-restraint, I did not drop that hammer.

Rather I emphasized that it was a decision for her and her alone, independent of what anyone else thought, and that she must quiet her chattering mind to make it.

Which in Steph's case is akin to asking a dog to drive.

For she has another serious addiction: the phone.

You can see her every day zipping around town in her bright red Mazda hatchback, a pretty blonde—hair wet as she hurtles from one commitment to another—yammering away on her BlackBerry.

As Dad said: "That car must run on lithium batteries. The phone has to be on for it to go."

When a profoundly emotional thing happens, Steph's style is to call scads of people and tell them about it. Which, I've witnessed firsthand, drives her crazy.

Last year, when Mom was near death, a distraught Steph would call several dozen people and tell them Mom was bleeding out after surgery and not likely to survive. Then Mom would rally, and Steph would have to call everyone back a day later.

Mom would have another near–death experience—a bowel obstruction—and Steph would burn up the minutes once again, then have to call everyone back when she rallied again.

"Steph, stop it! You're making yourself crazy. Let's just operate on a need-to-know basis."

On the ship, as we discussed searching for her birth mother, I suggested that she not call a host of friends and talk, talk, talk about looking for her.

"It does not matter what other people think," I told her. "Try weighing the pros and cons alone. In peace and quiet. Listen to what your soul is saying, and not the people around you."

That's our thing, I realize now. Something special be-tween the two of us. The thing fully realized on that trip.

Not traveling. Not adventure.

But being there for one another, so that we may unburden our hearts. Uncrowd our minds. And hear what our souls are saying.

In the six months since that trip, Steph and I have grown even closer. For months now, she has helped me dress, eat, brush, sit, stand, and walk.

She flew three hours with me recently to New York City, although she is panicked by flying and had not done so in years. She knew I could not manage a restroom without her.

I am kinda like having a two-year-old again. A two-year-old who smokes a lot. And God bless Stephanie—a respiratory therapist—for lighting me up without complaint.

"Just don't tell my students," she always says.

Not that Steph is always the most calm person I know, especially under pressure. Recently, she drove Marina and me to an appointment in my BMW, a car I bought for its keyless entry and push-button start after I could no long turn the key in the ignition of my van.

Steph drives me now, for I am no longer able. Usually, that's fine. But this time, she and Marina got out and closed their doors, forgetting where the key fob was: inside the car with me.

It was high noon on a summer day, and I was locked inside my black car with a black interior dressed in black. I couldn't reach in my pocket for the key, and couldn't lift my arms to unlock the doors. Like I said: a two-year-old.

What did Steph do? She freaked out. Tugged on the handle again and again, trying to magically open the locked door. Yelled and banged on the window. Looked around frantically for, I don't know . . . a rock to throw through the glass?

"Pipe down, missy!" I mouthed through the closed window. "Calm down! Stop!"

Poor Marina was trying to calm Stephanie, to no avail. My sister was wilting in the heat. She was so panicked, she wanted to call 911.

"Just wait," I said. "Calm down."

Sweat dripped in my eyes. I could not wipe it away. I focused. Scooted left in my seat, closer to the unlock button in the center of the dashboard. I leaned forward and mashed the button with my head.

Click! The locks popped open.

I rolled out "like a sausage," as Steph laughs when describing it now.

When we arrived home after the appointment, Steph locked me in the car again. And lost her mind again, just like the first time.

During another recent mishap, I was the one who lost my cool.

I had broken my left thumb—snapped accidentally as someone turned me over, unaware my bum thumb was extended. I was in bed resting when my sixty-pound dog Gracie stepped on said thumb. I wept.

Steph was trying to comfort me. I was so upset I couldn't tell her how I wanted my hand moved to relieve the pressure. Steph stood over me, flummoxed, weeping too.

You can tell a lot about a person by how they touch. And a lot of people now touch me, as they dress me and clean me and move me around.

I am constantly saying to others, "Careful. Slowly. Don't forget my thumb . . . ," or my legs, or whatever body part is flopping behind.

I am constantly telling Steph the opposite: scratch more fiercely, press firmer, pull harder. Her touch is too gentle.

She'll brush out my tangled hair delicately, like she's performing surgery. "Just yank the brush through!"

"Oh, I don't want to hurt you! You sure?"

"Darling, I would not suggest it if it hurt."

She strokes my head every time she moves hair out of my face.

She says, "I would do anything for you," and I believe her. I believe in her.

My children adore her. "Hello, sugar plums!" she greets them each time she sees them.

When Marina accidentally dyed a blond spot in the front of her hair, she asked Stephanie to fix it.

Wesley will sit on Steph's lap longer than any other human being's, including me. "Can I spend the night at your house?" he often asks her.

Aside from John, Stephanie is the one person on the planet I have absolute faith in to raise my children. I know she will love them like her own.

What providence that God gave me such a sister.

What peace of mind.

For me, sweet Steph, you are the greatest gift of all.

Everyone Should Keep a List of the Little Things They Love

(found on my iPhone, dated March 2012)

Smokin' hot 4-inch heels
The sexy feeling I get while wearing them
When Gracie licks my face
When no one is screaming at home
Starbucks chai tea latte skinny
Freesia: the smell, the colors
Lavender sunsets
Any sunset
The grace of an orchid
A chilled fine white wine
A friend to share it with
The silly feeling it leaves
Sitting by the dryer vent emitting fresh soapy air
Chinese potstickers, steamed not fried, with that soy-based
    sauce with little green onions
A beautifully iced cake that tastes as good as it looks
A handwritten letter from a friend
A steaming bath in a clawfoot tub
When my dog lies so close to me on the bed I can feel her heart
    beating
When my children do the same
A cup of coffee first thing in the morning. Cream and sugar
    please.
The song "Clair de Lune," because it reminds me of my sister
A pedicure when the lady rubs my feet and calves
When you can see rainbows in the sprinkler mist
When someone scratches my head for me

The Gift

April

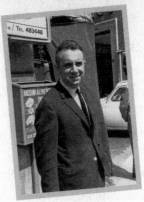

Panos

I n the late fall of 2009, while a series of doctors fumbled to figure out what was wrong with me, my mental detours started in force. My attempts to find some flippin' reason for my body's problems other than ALS.

My birth mother Ellen didn't help, as there was nothing wrong on her side.

That left my birth father.

In her second letter, Ellen had named him: Dr. Panos Kelalis. And in the next sentence, she told me she had heard through the grapevine that he was dead.

Dead.

Dead, dead, dead.

Dead.

I had never even considered the possibility.

Poof! Gone in one sentence was the chance to know him.

The chance to ask him why we are how we are.

The chance to say, "I am a part of you. And you a part of me."

I was angry, and I questioned Ellen's character. She had kept my birth father and me apart, unknown to each other. Had she only contacted me because he was dead? Because then she could dodge dealing with him and his family?

My thoughts were unkind. I had lost my birth father. And it hurt.

Don't focus on the loss, I told myself. Focus on the opportunity. The chance to explore the man he'd been.

Dr. Panos Kelalis. Dr. Panos Keh-LA-lease. For weeks, I turned the name over in my mind.

A doctor, as my mother always told me growing up. But I never quite believed her. Tee exaggerated many things. I mean, one semester of French, and *voilà!* Steph and I were fluent.

But my birth father really was a doctor.

And, by Jove, he really was Greek.

That had been the scourge of my childhood: my lack of ethnicity. My nondescript looks such a torment for my raven-haired Greek beauty mother.

No amount of Greek lessons, or performances of Greek traditional dances in little Greek outfits, would help. No amount of studying the Greek language with a bristly woman named Ms. Karadaras, who would pinch my ears if I didn't concentrate, would satisfy Theodora "Tee" Damianos. I just didn't look the part.

I was explaining this dynamic to a friend recently. It was something I had accepted years ago, but suddenly Stephanie, sitting beside me, started crying.

"It was never true," she said of our mother's criticisms. "It was never true. You were always so pretty."

"I didn't say pretty," I said in my slurred voice, trying to speak slowly and clearly. "I said I didn't think I was Greek."

Now I had my father's name. Panos Kelalis. As Greek as it gets.

I Googled away.

Dr. Kelalis was a surgeon.

Oh!

He worked for the prestigious Mayo Clinic, first in Minnesota, then Florida.

Oh!

He authored a seminal textbook for doctors in his field.

Oh!

His obituary in the Jacksonville, Florida, newspaper described him as an internationally renowned pioneer in pediatric urology.

In an instant, I felt so much smarter.

Gawd, I hope this is true, I thought.

As a journalist, I knew you could create a deceased person in your mind. Study his life. Define who he was. Create a feeling inside. Panos was dead, but not gone. I could re-create him in the things he left behind.

I requested a photo from the newspaper where his obituary appeared. It came, as all things seemed to, in a plain manila envelope. The next day, on my lunch break in a park, I opened it.

I stared at the gray-haired man in front of me.

These moments, when I first saw the faces of my birth parents, were not moments of blubbering. No crying out "Mama!" or "Papa!", a primal urge released. Rather, it was a studied calm. A stealthy search for my face in theirs.

I started with Panos's eyes. Our deep-set eyes, the ones that make me look like a raccoon if I put dark eyeshadow on.

I stared at the thick, skewer-straight eyebrows. Our eyebrows. Every time I had mine waxed, I said to the Vietnamese lady, "As much arch as possible, please," and she said, "I try! I try!" I would have one big straight caterpillar across my forehead if not for her.

I noticed our round cheeks, the ones my mother so criticized.

I smiled at our nose, with the slight bulb at the end. Not so bad if you look straight at it. But from a low angle, a fat mushroom. In 2010, there was a ginormous picture of me in the newspaper meeting my new dog Gracie. My head was tipped up as Gracie licked my face, and my God, my nose looked huge.

In his picture, thank goodness, Panos stared at me straight on.

I thought: What a handsome fellow.

Then caught myself.

Most of my adult life, I have looked at men in terms of whether I was attracted to them. I had long entered the phase where I loved gray hair.

I thought: Doh! You're not supposed to think he's handsome. That's your birth father.

Ahem. Okay. Distinguished, then. Panos looked so distinguished.

Near all my life, I had looked at the faces of the six Maass kids, my best friend Nancy's face most of all. I had marveled at the similarities. Memorized how they looked alike: who had their father's eyes, their mother's cheekbones, who got the dip in the chin.

Near all my life, I had looked upon my finely featured mother, and my handsome father, and couldn't find my face.

But in Panos's face, I saw myself.

Myself—in such an impressive man. A man, in that moment, I wanted to know everything about. I wanted him to come alive in that photo and speak to me, the daughter he never knew.

I started to reconstruct Panos as best I could. His obituary noted he had been married to a woman named Barbara. There was no mention of children.

Oh boy! I thought. What if all this happened after he was married?

I pictured some beautiful doctor's wife with a perfect life. Then me barging in and sullying a lifetime of memories with him.

No, please no.

I searched for a marriage certificate in Minnesota, since he worked at the Mayo Clinic in Rochester when I was conceived.

Nothing.

I checked the public records of Jacksonville, Florida, where he last lived, and found court records.

The state of Florida leads the United States in open-records laws. Lawsuits, arrest reports, divorces, even wills, are public domain.

My domain. As a court reporter, I had used these records for years.

I found Panos's probate records. I saw there was ongoing litigation over his estate. There was a certificate of death, but no cause of death listed.

And there was a will, a spare document with three trustees: Robert Abdalian, Soulla Economides, and Stelios Iannou.

How the hell do you even pronounce that? I thought. And how do I locate them?

Only one name had a quick-click Google answer. There was a Stelios Iannou Foundation in Cyprus. Panos had left most of his estate to disabled children. Awesome. And not just disabled children, but the disabled children of Cyprus.

My birth father was a Greek Cypriot.

I brought the globe to my desk and spun it around. There was Cyprus, a small island in the Mediterranean, south of Turkey and west of Syria and Lebanon.

Cyprus, I thought. How unexpected.

How cool.

I wondered if I might have some mysterious illness that only affected Greek Cypriots. Jewish folks suffer Tay-Sachs, black folks sickle-cell anemia. Perhaps on Cyprus—population about 1.4 million—they suffered something too.

I wrote a lawyer in Jacksonville, one of a few listed on Panos's court documents. No response. So I called.

"Were you Panos's lawyer?" I asked.

"No, I am the lawyer for one of the lawyers," he said.

Oh Lord, I thought.

I told the lawyer I was a daughter Panos never knew of and wanted to contact the trustees or relatives to ask for medical history.

The lawyer was like "Suuuurrrrre!" and totally blew me off.

Dead end.

Then my extraordinary pal Nancy struck again.

You see, Nancy never forgets a friend. And is such a generous and helpful soul, she naturally assumes this in others. Which is to say, Nancy not only thought of a man we had both known twenty years ago, but thought nothing of asking for his help.

"Call George!" Nancy said.

George Sycallides. A fellow graduate student in the journalism program at the University of Florida. An international student from—I had forgotten!—Cyprus.

I found George, dusted off the little Greek I knew, and spoke to him on the phone.

"*Yassou! Ti kanis?* Man, George, have I got a story for you!"

George listened intently. "Really? Really?" he said over and over.

I asked for a favor: Could he contact the two trustees I believed were in Cyprus, Soulla Economidou and Stelios Iannou?

"Of course, Susan. Of course," he said

I was hoping he would simply locate Soulla and Stelios and see if they spoke English. Then I would contact them.

George called back within days. Stelios was dead, George said, but Soulla was alive. She was Panos's cousin. "I told her everything!" George said merrily.

Yes, George was telling Soulla about a nurse at the Mayo Clinic who had a baby girl . . . when Soulla broke in: "Panos has a daughter?"

"She would be thrilled to meet you!" George said.

Good old George. Talk about kicking open a door!

I sent an e-mail to Soulla, emphasizing my mysterious illness and that I sought only medical information. George gave me an address, and I sent pictures of my family. Close-ups, where Soulla could see features clearly.

Soulla opened one photo and was stunned.

Not a photo of me, but of my little cocoa-bean son with hazel eyes. The one who tans up like me, unlike my blue-eyed kids who burn like their dad.

My son Aubrey looked exactly like my birth father.

Three weeks later, on February 19, 2010, I received an e-mail from Soulla, via her daughter Alina in London.

"When George called me," she wrote, "after a while I felt like it was Christmas and I had a present I never expected. You are so welcome. I have two daughters (Alina and Mania) and two granddaughters (Phaedra and Anastasia) and Avraam (my son-in-law). I have many photos of Panos. In one especially (he was about 6 years old) he looks exactly like you! The ears are absolutely identical! Can't wait to see you."

Alina assured me that "everything mum writes in her brief note to you is heartfelt from all of us here :-)."

Would it have happened without George? I don't know.

But I can never thank him enough for his role.

In April 2010, I arrived in Cyprus. It was less than two months since I corresponded with Soulla. Less than five months since, through a court order, I had my adoption papers unsealed on health grounds and found out that Panos Kelalis was officially listed as my father. Less than eight months since I noticed the withering in my left hand.

No time to waste.

I wanted to know.

If this book is about the journeys I took because of my ALS, then this was the first. A journey into my birth father's past and forward into his relatives' present.

I previously described seeing a picture of Ellen for the first time as staring into the sun. My personal sun. A recognition so bright it blinded me.

Cyprus would too.

I had never considered finding my birth father. Never. Now a turn of fate, and here I was on an airplane, zipping across Europe on the edge of an Icelandic volcanic explosion. Traveling to meet a dozen people I didn't know. To introduce myself, the illegitimate daughter of a dead man they had long admired. Writing my own life and rewriting his.

I couldn't get my head around it, much less my heart. I needed someone with me to pinch me, to witness the unreal and tell me it was true. That person, as always, was Nancy.

A public relations pro, Nancy would have made a fine journalist. She remembers things so precisely. Every detail. Every foible. Each time she tells a story, it's loaded with minutiae most people forget.

You know those cars outfitted with 360-degree cameras that drive around mapping streets for Google?

It's like Nancy does that in her head.

Nancy journaled while we were in Cyprus. The puff of air freshener at the doctor's office, the off-color joke of a cousin—she noted it all.

She kept me grounded and focused on the details: the purple flowers that never wilted, dead or alive. The seasoning on the souvlaki. The tang of salt in the dry Mediterranean air.

I was overwhelmed when meeting Panos's family. Nancy carried the conversations for me, spoke when I was too moved to speak, brought presents that I had not thought to bring.

She helped me see the beauty of Cyprus. Warm. Fresh and sunny like the Mediterranean of our dreams, with terraced buildings and rocky outcroppings. A dry tropical oasis, unlike the lush mugginess of Florida.

But cultivated. Orange trees. Palms. Bougainvillea. The handiwork of a dozen cultures over a thousand years that had made this island home.

A crossroads. "A lifeboat for the Middle East," as Soulla's son-in-law Avraam described it to me. An old place. A place to dig and dig and always find something new.

Thank heavens for George. He set up the whole trip and sent us a daily schedule in advance. He made appointments to meet Soulla and other relatives. Told us exactly where to go, and when, and offered his house as a home base.

"Welcome Nancy and Suzin," read a sign when we arrived, a high-hanging banner made by his eight-year-old son Stelios.

George's home was outside the Cypriot capital, Nicosia, a contemporary white abode in the middle of a golden wheat field. For me, those are the colors of the Cyprus: white and gold. Like the sun.

And blue, like the Mediterranean. So many shades of blue.

We had a fish dinner, straight from the sea, and wine. George was, as he joked in one of our first e-mail exchanges, "still the dashing, bright, handsome male you knew at UF but with less hair due to . . . maturity reasons." We talked into the night with him and his wife Yioula, drinking wine long after the fish was finished.

After dinner, George brought out an extensive family tree of Panos's relatives. He had included everyone he could find. It was six sheets of paper, taped together. He rattled off the names of the people he had spoken with, telling me details. The tree listed more than sixty people, but that night it seemed like six hundred.

Including me.

There I was, on a short branch in the splay of Greek names like Petrides, Georgiades, Michaelides. My plain-Jane name, "Susan Spencer," among the -ides and -ios and -is.

I was overjoyed.

But that night, I turned the family tree over in my mind. Wondering. Was I really one of them?

Panos had no descendants or immediate family . . . except me. But as is common in Greek culture, he had been close with his aunts and uncles and cousins. And the person he had perhaps been closest with, from childhood onward, was his cousin Soulla.

Soulla had been kind to me over e-mail, referring to me as the unexpected gift. But I couldn't help but wonder, would she like the gift as much when she opened it? What would she think when she actually met me?

Would I live up to the legacy of my birth father?

The next day we drove into the heart of Nicosia, a city of contrasts. An ancient walled area, near high-rise buildings. Crisp Mediterranean architecture in hills miles from the sea. A European feel with strong Middle Eastern influences. Sleepy but alive, crowded but compact, familiar but comfortably foreign.

Soulla's apartment was in a modern building on a busy

street. I smiled when I saw the name: Attikus Street. Wesley's first name is Atticus.

We took a private elevator to her floor. George, who had visited her already, said it opened right into her apartment.

Soulla was a widow. Her husband might have been elected president of Cyprus, her children told us, if he had not died. I had worn black, out of courtesy for her status, halfway expecting a four-foot-nine stooped babushka clad in mourning black from head-to-toe.

Then Soulla opened the door, dressed in jeans and a T-shirt.

"Hi! Hello! I have been excited all day!" she said.

We stepped into her apartment, a wide open, light-filled space, with stained glass lamps and antiques, built-in display cases full of tidy collections, and artwork, including her daughter Alina's icon paintings, framed in a zinging electric blue.

The home of an aristocrat, yet perfectly comfortable.

Just like Soulla.

We sat outside on her terrace. I studied the lines of the buildings around us, a jumble of apartments with hills beyond. Soulla studied my face. Subtly. Searching for Panos. Torn between maintaining a polite gaze and staring.

She ordered souvlaki from a local restaurant. It was delivered with a bright salad of tomatoes and cukes. (We should have this in America. Where is the souvlaki delivery van?) We ate and talked all evening.

Soulla is an affluent, educated, tiny woman, maybe a hundred pounds after a large meal. Her English was perfect, her conversation effortless. She exuded warmth and thoughtfulness, as natural as any woman on the street, not a stroke of makeup or whit of snobby air despite her upper-class status.

It was apparent, immediately and often, that she had loved and admired Panos, her older cousin. Loved how Panos was tenderhearted with patients. How he was always loyal and kind. How he adored her children.

Soulla talks with her hands, her gestures revealing as much as her words. She has one where she says, "It was . . . ," and drifts off, shaking her hand, shrugging her shoulders, closing her eyes, and inhaling deeply, signaling something divine.

"To know he had a daughter . . . ," she said, and gestured just so.

She explained their devastation when Panos died suddenly in 2002. He had flown back to Cyprus for the birth of Soulla's first granddaughter. He felt ill after the flight, and went to bed. He never woke up.

Soulla said my sudden appearance in their lives was like a piece of him returned. A gift. "Like Christmas," she said again, gesturing just so.

Soulla showed me pictures of Panos. There he was sitting in a café in Italy, in his twenties, his profile just like mine. There he was as a child, his wingnut ears and eyes exactly like Aubrey's.

He was fearless.

That's what Soulla kept saying. Panos was fearless.

He would help anyone. Go anywhere. Face any challenge.

Months later, Panos's best friend Robert Abdalian would tell me how Panos would swim way into the ocean, out of sight of the shore. Bob used the same word: fearless.

I took the word into my soul. Fearless was in my genes.

After a while, Soulla's daughter Mania came by. She lived in the same building. A mother like me, with two girls I would meet later, Anastasia—pronounced the elegant Greek way, AH na-sta-SI-ah—and Phaedra.

Another hour, and Mania's husband, Avraam—the operator, as I always thought of him—arrived with a bottle of wine.

Avraam was quiet the first few days, but after that, he was nonstop. He later told me my sudden appearance panicked him. He wondered if he too might have a daughter he didn't know about. "From college, you know."

As I said, an operator.

Avraam is a business engineer. Here's how he explains this in his e-mail signature line: "BUSINESS ENGINEERING involves industrial & environmental management, innovation management, entrepreneurship, marketing engineering, services management, operational research, econometrics, global strategy and leadership, management science, business administration, finance, economics, mathematics, social science (ethics and law)."

And as Avraam will unabashedly tell you, he's an expert in each subject.

He brought the electric car to Cyprus, he told me. I ordered a Red Bull one day in front of him. "I brought Red Bull to Cyprus!" he said.

Like them all, Avraam adored Panos. "He had an unbelievable rationality," Avraam told me that first evening. "He was no BOOL-sheeter."

He poured the last of the wine, went for another bottle. Soulla kept showing me pictures, talking about Panos. As the wine went around, the talk cycled into Greek. Despite a childhood of Saturdays spent with Ms. Karadaras pinching my ears, I couldn't understand a word. It sounded like Russians speaking Italian to me.

And yet I felt at home.

Eventually, Soulla would show me a fifty-something-year-old family photo, maybe twenty people, including Panos's parents, aunts, and uncles. I got out my reporter's notebook and asked her to name each person.

Something -ios. Some-other-person -ides.

"And who is this gentleman?" I asked, pointing to a swarthy, stocky figure in black.

"That would be your grandmother," Soulla said.

Grandmother Julia, Soulla explained, had been blessed with brains, not looks. She had been a mustachioed woman. So much so, according to Alina, she had scared the grandchildren.

We laughed and laughed about this, Soulla included.

It was perfect. Levity and gravity, at the same time.

The next morning, Soulla took me to meet the doctor, a friend, who had pronounced Panos dead. There had been no autopsy, but the doctor assured me Panos had no neurological problems that would explain my withered hand. He had died of something vascular—likely an aneurysm—after the long flight, the doctor opined.

Phew! I thought. Still no sign of hereditary ALS.

Soulla confirmed it: no known genetic problems in her family.

In fact, she and Panos had a hundred-year-old cousin. Xenon, the centenarian, was in excellent health. A doctor himself, he had helped Panos with his career. Soula arranged for Nancy, George, and me to meet him.

Cousin Nadia accompanied us. Nadia is similar to Soulla: tiny, tasteful, in her sixties. But Nadia is a spitfire, prone to off-color jokes. A professional interpreter of Greek, Italian, and English, she once had a chance to translate during a visit by the pope. She declined. "I never really liked the man," she said.

It was a short climb up stairs to Xenon's apartment—something that bothered us when we found out that Xenon was in a wheelchair and hadn't been able to leave the apartment for years.

Xenon met us in his living room. He had a blue blazer on over his pajamas. His hearing aid stuck out of its breast pocket.

His much younger wife, Irini (only in her eighties), joined us.

Xenon had been Cyprus's minister of health. He told us how he had worked with Lord Mountbatten, eradicating malaria. How both his sons were doctors. How he had practiced medicine around the world.

In his youth, he had typhoid. Typhoid! Xenon was in the middle of that story when Irini, his silent wife, finally barked, "SHE WANTS TO HEAR ABOUT PANOS!"

"He can tell stories till tomorrow," Irini said, shaking her head.

This got Nancy, Nadia, and me giggling.

Undeterred, Xenon went on. "Before the war . . . " he started.

And George politely broke in: "WHICH WAR?"

He shouted, of course, because Xenon couldn't hear. Which made Nancy, Nadia, and me giggle harder. George looked horrified.

Nadia asked if Irini had pictures of Panos. The two disappeared to another room and returned with scads of framed photos.

"Of her boys, the doctors!" Nadia said, rolling her eyes.

Laugh. Smile. It was a delightful afternoon, even if I didn't learn much about my birth father. Except for one precious, ethereal detail.

As we left, I leaned and gave Xenon a kiss on each cheek, the Cypriot custom.

"Ah!" the old man said, smiling. "You kiss like Panos."

I have always loved Greek food—stuffed grape leaves, sharp feta cheese, ink-black olives steeped in rosemary and garlic.

In Cyprus, I discovered the best way to eat: at a mezze. A word from the Arabic meaning "to share," a mezze was a variety of courses, shared by all at the table, common throughout the Middle East. A reminder that a meal is more than food.

Early in the trip, we shared a seafood mezze courtesy of the spitfire Nadia. It included every type of shellfish, roe, octopus, and urchin, filleted fishes large and small, served on white plates upon white linen. Delight.

Near the end, in a small tavern with russet walls and deep brown tables, we shared an unforgettable meat mezze with Soulla's extended family. It was Soulla's gift, though she was a vegetarian herself.

First came quail eggs and marinated artichokes, sauteed mushrooms, warm pita with hummus and spicy caponata.

Then course after course of meats: souvlaki, roasted chicken, pork in all varieties, followed by lamb in a mint-reduction sauce. Spinach pie. Moussaka with a toasted top of savory custard. Couscous with broth. Vegetables.

And desserts. Cinnamon-cheese pastries, honey-laden phyllo dough vessels full of ground pistachios.

We lingered over each course. Each offering. Each bite. We talked and laughed, whiling away hours.

Eventually, we moved outside for the evening's final coffee and nightcap. The night sky was clear. The world close and warm. No shadows between us.

Mania remarked to Nancy on our friendship. "It's not something that can ever be re-created," Nancy replied, crying.

Avraam, who didn't understand the grim specter of my health, asked questions. I cried as I explained it might be ALS, a death sentence.

"But . . . " I eked out, "no matter what happens, I am fortunate. I have met all of you. I can tell my children: 'You are not sentenced by genes to suffer.'

"I now know that part of me came from a great man. And great people."

I talked of the parents who adopted me. Who sacrificed for me. Who expected great things for me, stood by me, and made me who I am.

I said I felt like the luckiest person in the world.

And I did.

I might have been dying, but that night—on that terrace,

after that meal, with those people—I was experiencing the full wonder of life.

I had arrived a stranger, but I was leaving with a new family.

I was unafraid.

Fearless.

I carried those feelings home with me, along with an antique bracelet—a gift from Soulla, exactly the kind I would have bought myself—and two cherished possessions found on Panos's body when he died: his rosary and his Saint Andreas medallion.

I had the medallion mounted on onyx. I wear it often as a necklace, close to my heart.

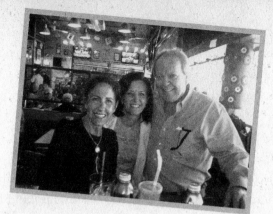

The Bible

Two years later, my trip to Cyprus still resonated in my soul. Among my relatives I had found no answers, but I had found peace. I had felt accepted, as I rarely had before.

Even though I had never known Panos, it was the land of my heritage. My second home.

I wanted to return. To take John, introduce him around, and hear him assure me that he understood. That he would take the children there one day to meet their relatives.

I wanted to thank Soulla and her family.

To finish what I had started and discover more of the man my birth father had been.

I wanted to return in the spring. The cruise with Stephanie was in March. I was saving the summer for my children, when they would be out of school. That left two months for Cyprus.

But Nadia, my spitfire cousin, had been diagnosed with

cancer and was in the middle of chemotherapy. Then Soulla had spinal surgery, which necessitated a long convalescence. The trip would have to be delayed until June.

No bother. I still had time.

And one important thing to do for Soulla before I returned.

To get her a gift as dear as the ones she gave me.

In Cyprus, it was clear that Panos's family had no love for Barbara, the American woman Panos had married—and divorced—and married again. And divorced a second time.

Barbara was "a spoiled American princess," they said. She had hissy fits at restaurants. Refused to participate in events if she was mad at Panos or someone else.

Each time they said her name—ruefully—they precisely pronounced each syllable BAR-ba-ra: "BAR-ba-ra was difficult!" Panos's nephew-in-law Avraam said, circling a finger around an ear.

The final insult, according to Soulla, was when she asked BAR-ba-ra to bring the family Bible back to Cyprus for Panos's funeral, and she had not.

"If you meet her and see the Bible—grab it!" Soulla said to me, partly in jest. Words I never forgot.

I became determined to get that Bible for Soulla.

And to meet BAR-ba-ra. I mean, Panos had married and divorced her twice? I was fascinated. Must have been one helluva love.

So I wrote BAR-ba-ra in Jacksonville, Florida, where she and Panos last lived. The letter returned unopened. A dead end. I needed help.

I thought of Pat McKenna. Pat is a nationally known

private investigator, having worked for the defense in O. J. Simpson's murder trial, William Kennedy Smith's rape case, and Casey Anthony's murder trials.

I had met Pat a decade before on a lower-profile case. A mother had left her toddler sleeping at home while she picked up a present nearby on tony Worth Avenue in Palm Beach.

The two-year-old had woken up and drowned in their backyard pool. The rest of the press pilloried her, partially because of the nature of the errand.

I believed as a mom that it was immaterial whether the woman left the child to buy Louis Vuitton luggage or a gallon of milk. She left the child. That was the crime.

Pat thanked me at the end of the case for being fair.

Pat and I hadn't spoken much since. We were Facebook friends, though, so I sent him a private message.

I deliberated how dramatic I should make it and thought, Ah, why not? It is what it is.

I wrote:

> Dear Pat,
> I would like to hire you to find somebody. It's a dying wish . . .

He showed up at my front door the next day, offering his services for free. Later, he told me he hadn't even noticed the "dying wish" part. He just wanted to help me if he could.

Now, Pat is a charmer. His premier investigative skill is talking to people. The man could talk a cat out of a box of mice. He also uses the saltiest damn language of any human I know.

"I was on the balls of my ass too!" he said, explaining how he had been flat broke when a tabloid newspaper offered him a million bucks to spill secret details of O. J.'s murder case.

Pat turned the offer down.

He spares no salty spite for people who opine on Casey Anthony while sitting at computers in their dirty underwear. But he phrases that in a far more crass way.

Yes, Pat's remarkably crude.

"I'll either charm it out of her or intimidate it out of her," Pat said, when I explained about Barbara. "I'll give her a dirt nap if she doesn't give you that Bible!"

But also remarkably dear.

When he phoned BAR-ba-ra the first time—it seemed to take him about five minutes to find her with a database search—Pat had to step away from me to regain his composure, choking up as he explained to her my health.

Barbara, for her part, was completely unaware of my existence.

And completely disbelieving.

She was so embroiled with lawyers and legal issues involving Panos's estate, even ten years after his death, that she mistook our call to be an offshoot of that.

"No ma'am," Pat said. "Susan has no interest in the estate. She wants nothing of you except information about Panos and his family Bible, if you would be so kind."

They hung up. Soon came a call from Barbara's protective older brother, an elderly man from Texas.

Now, you must understand, Texas is a unique state with a rebel spirit all its own, the one I imagine most likely to secede from the United States if given the chance.

Texas is so large it has its own power grid—one of only three in the United States: one for the eastern half, one for the western half, and one for Texas.

And this guy had an oversize Texas personality. The man once sued Panos, his own brother-in-law. That's how brash they are in Texas.

He had choice words for Pat and me, spoken in a Texas twang so thick my ears rang. "I hear you're harassin' my sister," he growled.

Barbara, he said, had had a heart attack and a stroke. "You're gonna kill her. My friend is running for top prosecutor, and I'm helping him get elected. He says you could get charged with accessory to murder. I would hate for you to get charged or sued."

Bring it on! I thought.

He twanged on about how Panos couldn't have fathered a child because he was made sterile after an accident in the early 1960s. Now, he could tell me Panos's penis got cut off and launched into space, and I would still believe he was my birth father. So I was not one scrap deterred by his threats.

Of course, Pat wasn't either.

Pat spoke gingerly to him, promised to send him photos and records, and asked him to reconsider when he got them.

"Fuckin' hillrod," Pat said as we hung up, using his own word combo of *hillbilly* and *nimrod*.

In the following days, Pat fielded long calls from a curious Barbara, convincing her to meet us. Barbara did not believe I was Panos's daughter, but she was willing to give me the Bible if it brought me comfort.

Soon after, Pat, Nancy, and I flew to meet her in Knoxville, Tennessee, where she had just moved. It was my first airplane trip using a wheelchair. Another milestone crossed.

I thought of how Nancy and I had joked and joked about this mythical woman. Laughed about how we might have to dress in all-black and burgle her home to get the Bible—committing a sin, a crime, and an act of love at the same time.

I thought of how, out of gratitude, I should erase from my mind all the disparaging things we had heard of Barbara. She had been kind.

That afternoon, Barbara came to our hotel. Her lady helper drove her there in a big green Mercedes. Pat helped her in. She used an elegant cane, the only indicator that she was well into her seventies, at least.

Her hair was a deep brown, setting off her eyes, a crystal blue. Her skin was flawless. She smelled like roses.

"Nice to meet you," she said, sitting near me and taking my near-lifeless hand. "How was your flight?"

She held the Bible in her free hand.

As she talked of Panos, her blue eyes widened and took on a dreamy look. "He and I, we were one."

She was a remarkably beautiful woman.

And exceedingly polite. She did not pepper me with questions, nor stare. She invited us to dinner. I could tell by the way she specified a certain seat in the restaurant and ordered off the menu she was a particular lady.

I thought of how hard it was for her to learn that a man she thought was uniquely hers was not. She had moved to Knoxville, where she knew no one, which I thought odd and sad. I felt sorry for her.

That night she handed me the Bible.

Back in the hotel room, Nancy, Pat, and I checked it out. Nancy was the first one to say it: "Doesn't look like a family Bible to me!"

Nancy described her own family's Bible, a huge tome in German that had had its own stand, its pages crumbling with age.

The Bible Barbara had given me looked unused. It was a standard size in English, with a wood cover engraved with a Greek Orthodox cross. We checked the publication date: 1957.

Pat 'fessed up that he had spotted a religious bookstore near the hotel. "We've been had!" Pat concluded. "Fuckin' hill-rods!" He started anew on his I'll-give-her-a-dirt-nap rant.

"Calm down, people," I said. "We can talk more with her at her house tomorrow."

Nancy messaged the folks in Cyprus to try to get a description of the family Bible. My iPhone chimed before dawn. It was Soulla. Nancy spoke to her.

As I stirred awake, I heard Nancy asking for a description of the Bible, then saying: "Whaaaat??? You don't know?"

As it turned out, Soulla had not seen the Bible since childhood. She said the only person who could identify it was Xenon, the then hundred-year-old cousin we'd met two years before.

"He's still alive?" Nancy blurted out.

When Pat joined us, we gave him the good and bad news. Good that there was someone who could check the Bible's authenticity. Bad that the person was . . . not so reliable.

"Lemme get this straight," Pat said. "Our bona fide is one hundred and two years old?"

"Yup!" we said, laughing.

We vowed to case Barbara's house for the real-deal Bible when we visited her that day.

We lunched with Barbara at a wonderful place, the North-shore Brasserie. I remember two things from the meal: (1) The ice cream. Handmade. Caramel lime. Best I've ever had. (2) A breakthrough with Barbara.

At the meal, I brought up the story of my birth mother. Barbara, I realized, was too polite or nervous to ask. I was not spot-on sure about the dates of her relationship with Panos, or whether I had been conceived while they were . . . ugh . . . married.

I eased her into a conversation about how they met. She was a patient in the hospital where he worked. And when they married. 1967.

Phew!!!!

Well after my conception.

I asked Barbara to remember that the pregnancy—that I—had happened before Panos met her. "All this does not detract from what the two of you had," I said to her. I saw her blue eyes widen with recognition and relief.

We went to her house, a huge home even by American standards, in an upscale Knoxville suburb. A home where she lived alone.

Barbara tottered up the steps to her towering front doors. Pat helped us both in. He was so helpful the whole trip. I was using a wheelchair off and on, and he lugged it around. I heard him groan one day as he hoisted it into the car trunk. "There goes a seminal vesicle!" he said cheerily.

The man was an absolute gentleman when he wanted to be. He even tucked away his F-bombs for Barbara. She was too much a lady (unlike me) to find them amusing.

Barbara's home was decorated in Baroque style, with lots of gold accents and fine furniture. Formal, like Barbara. She had a trio of tiny dogs. Their yips echoed through the house.

We sat. I realized that I had never seen Panos's handwriting.

Can you tell something about a person by his handwriting? I can.

I asked Barbara if I might see letters he had written to her. I cringe now, thinking of how nervy this was: I was asking to see their most private communication.

I never saw them.

But oh! what I did see.

Barbara brought out newspaper clippings of Panos's many accomplishments at the Mayo Clinic. Stories of patients saved. Awards won. Books written and charities supported.

We sat in her fancy living room, with near floor-to-ceiling windows all around, both of us reading the articles. It was so sunny, I squinted in the light.

At one point, Barbara stopped talking. I looked up. She was staring at me.

"You are squinting just like Panos," Barbara said.

In that moment, she believed.

She brought out some antique icons that had belonged to Panos. She laid them out in front of me. "Take whatever you wish," she said. I chose one.

She gave me the gold worry beads that Panos thumbed.

The gold money clip found in Panos's pocket when he died, the euros still in it. No, I never counted them. There could be hundreds, but I would never spend them.

Pat and Nancy asked about the Bible. Barbara said it was the only one she had.

Nancy wandered the large home. She had asked the Cyprus relatives about other items, and they mentioned a painting of an ocean scene by a prominent Greek artist that Panos had owned and loved. Nancy was hell's-bells intent on finding that painting too.

Barbara had recently moved in. Some things were still boxed, some pictures not yet hung. Nancy saw an ocean painting, but it looked too poorly done to be the one that had stirred Panos's soul.

She spotted another painting, Mediterranean in color and feel, and brought it out to Barbara and me. That's Nancy. So stylish and professional, my good-girl friend, but she always took things a step further. Pushed me to explore more, to seek more. To ask. To try.

Yes, the painting was the one Panos had loved. Barbara offered it to me.

She was so kind. She kissed me on the way out, smelling like roses. I felt badly leaving her alone in that large house, no doubt longing for the love she once had.

Panos's relatives considered it cuckoo for him to marry and divorce her twice. Panos's best friend, Bob Abdalian, no fan of Barbara's either, told me he believed Panos viewed her like a patient, trying to help her.

But I know there was more. I saw her beauty, when others did not.

I find it extraordinary that he had as much patience for her as he did.

I have no idea why they never had children. There are things even nervy me won't ask. But they didn't. And now Barbara is alone.

Perhaps that's why she called me "stepdaughter" and shared so much.

The painting she gave me now hangs in the room where I sometimes sleep. My father hung it there without asking a single question about it.

It is of the ocean. Blue and green waves churning, a white froth atop them, sun glinting off the surface.

It is often the last thing I see before falling asleep.

The
Chickee
Hut

May

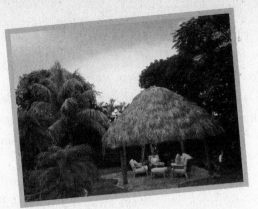

A Place of My Own

I
n many ways, my father Tom and I have a distant relationship. All through my childhood, he worked ten
hours a day at his pharmacy, six days a week. On Sunday, he was at church. He was working for us, I know, but I
missed him.

I used to lie awake at night, watching for the headlights of
his car to pull into the driveway at nine or ten o'clock. Many
times I fell asleep by the nightlight in the hallway, waiting for
him to return.

I loved when he let me haul away the branches after he
trimmed our ficus hedge, because yard work was one of the
few things we did together.

I worshipped my dad as a child. He was always kind to
me.

As adults, though, we seemed to grow further apart. The
distance was intractable, really, for he never talked. In the
twenty-five years before Mom got sick, I don't think Dad

called me five times. He lived one mile away, but never asked me to have lunch or see a movie with him.

But Dad remained kind. He picked up my kids when I was working, and he picks them up now that I am too sick to drive. He runs errands for me. He takes the boys for scooter rides.

Dad is a handyman extraordinaire. He can build or fix just about anything, and always assured us he was happy to do so. He built bunk beds for the boys. Bookshelves for me. Mounted crown molding in all our rooms.

That was my father's love language, I eventually realized: doing, not saying.

When I was well, I flitted in and out of my house, noticing the kids' clothes strewn about, the crusted dishes in the sink, the hair in the shower drain.

Oh, well, I thought, such is life.

But when I became sick, I started to notice bigger things. Or maybe the little things seemed bigger.

Like the chipped paint on the gutters. The dull walls that needed a "Pop!" The dilapidated dining table (a dump site for clean laundry) abused for years by kids, including one who drew on it with a Sharpie.

I called Dad.

"I'd sure love to have a built-in bench in the dining area—with storage," I said. "And, oh! a built-in entertainment center on the opposite wall."

"Okay. Just give me a drawing," Dad said.

"But we probably should paint the ceiling first."

"Who?" he said.

Said ceiling was twelve feet high, with tongue-in-groove

wood planks and beams. It would have to be brush-painted by hand, not rolled or sprayed.

"You, Dad! There's no one better!"

So Dad did it. Cheerfully. Stood atop a ladder for days at seventy-three years old, head crooked, painting the ceiling as I barked color orders.

"Super white on beams! White white on planks!"

We never said anything about my withered hand, or the doctor's appointments that ended in questions, not answers. We had only awkward silence about my illness. Even after my diagnosis in June, Dad never gave consolation or inspiration. He never acknowledged that I was sick.

But he gave me that gorgeous white ceiling.

It's funny what a difference a coat of paint can make.

After my diagnosis, John and I hired professionals to paint our house tan with a coral accent. Afterward, Dad stood in the blazing Florida sun, painting all our poolside French doors a deep navy blue.

I took two old sailfish mounts to a taxidermist to be refurbished. One was a six-footer Mom and Dad hooked in 1962. The other came from a neighbor's garbage.

We hung the sailfish by the blue doors. "Pop!"

I realize now what I was doing: I was nesting. Creating a dream home. The one I wanted to spend my last years in. The one I wanted to leave behind for my husband and kids.

As the cooler weather of the south Florida winter took hold, I began to spend much of my time outside: writing, planning trips and projects, smoking my cigs, more it seemed each day. Steering clear of the general hubbub of television and trumpet practice and arguing kids.

I sat for months underneath a canvas awning on our cement pool deck in a folding director's chair, staring out at our lovely yard. I watched the mangos plump up more each day. I admired the wide variety of palms.

That is another story of my parents' goodness. A friend and former neighbor, Bart, is a botanist, nursery owner, and landscaper. Years ago, he landscaped our entire front yard for free. Why?

"I just want to do something for you and your parents. They were so good to me," Bart said.

He heard of my diagnosis and offered to landscape the backyard as well. Bart took me to his nursery, and we picked a slew of mature trees that otherwise would have cost thousands.

There were triangle palms, coconut palms, spindle palms, banana palms, and bottle palms, the single, double, and triple variety. There was a prized rare bush palm he was so proud of. I can't remember its name, only the goodness of its gift.

(I just looked it up. A dwarf palmetto palm. Thank you, Bart!)

He helped us plant them around the edges of our pool deck and yard. I sat underneath the awning each day, enjoying them. Enjoying life.

That is one of the glories of south Florida: sitting outside in shorts surrounded by palms.

Then the heat arrived, radiating up from the cement deck and contained by the awning. Even in shade, it was like sitting in an Easy-Bake oven.

One day it was so hot, I saw a mirage on our wide-open lawn: a cool oasis. Perhaps a pergola or a covered porch? Or . . . my brain locked on to . . . a Chickee hut.

Aka, a tiki hut.

An open-air hut, no sides, with a high palm-frond roof. Florida's Miccosukee Indians had long built Chickee huts for housing. The high roof was waterproof and didn't absorb heat, creating a cool, shaded spot.

Many people build bars under Chickee huts. I envisioned a big, comfy seating area, with teak furniture, cushioned sofas, tables, pillows, candles, ottomans, a place John and I could gather friends and enjoy life.

A place where our children and their friends could hang out, not under our noses, but under our watch.

I pitched the Chickee idea to John.

"No. I like the open yard," he said.

I began wearing him down. "Man, these director's chairs are uncomfortable!"

"Man, it's hot out here!"

"Think of it as a vacation destination in our own back-yard!"

He wouldn't budge.

He was concerned about money, and the project creating more work for him. He was already overworked.

"Won't hurt to get an estimate," I said. "And I will do everything, I promise."

This was early May. By then, typing on my iPad was near impossible. My hands grew too tired on the large keyboard. My fingers and palm dragged over the touchscreen.

I would aim my curled, quivering finger like a sharp-shooter over the letter and hope to hell I hit target.

Hello iPhone!

Its tiny touchscreen keyboard was perfect, because I

still had one helluva right thumb. With that thumb on the iPhone, I have written one hundred thousand words the same way you would write a text message. I wrote near this entire book that way.

And I used that thumb to find a contractor and punch up a Chickee estimate.

The estimate was reasonable. We could afford it. I proceeded full-bore. Didn't wait for John's approval, which annoyed him.

"Please involve me in decisions," he texted me from work.

"Okay. Sorry."

John agreed to everything, but with one caveat: the Chickee would have to be built toward the back of the yard, close to the fence and property line, to maintain some open space in the middle of the yard.

"Agreed," I said.

Friends helped me gather the permits, complete them, and contact the Chickee builder.

We live in a small, tidy suburb in the middle of West Palm Beach called Lake Clarke Shores. The town is full of nice homes and has lots of legal codes about where things can be built.

I call the enforcers the "code cabal," but the rules do make for a nice community—large homes with ample open space around them. You are not allowed to build anything too close to the property lines in Lake Clarke, including where John wanted the Chickee.

We would have to apply for a variance, which would take two months and cost hundreds more. I was already living by a stopwatch. "Please, John, just agree to put it in the middle of yard. Think of it as less lawn to mow. Please."

"Okay," he relented.

A Chickee hut, fourteen by sixteen feet, got underway. First four poles were sunk in three feet of concrete. Then atop them a skeleton structure of cedar beams.

Then came fronds by the truckload. Thousands of them. Fronds of the sabal palm, which cannot be torn and repel water. Their large fan shape is folded and stapled flush, twelve layers in all.

The mirage came to life before my eyes.

I tapped on my iPhone and bought teak furniture: two sofas and two chairs. "You can do more damage with that one thumb than I can with all my faculties," John said.

Next to the fabric shop, helped by friends, for the perfect upholstery and pillows. Just so happened a weatherproof fabric called Sunbrella was on sale in a delightful soft orange called Mango Bubble. Perfect!

We wired the hut for electric—what's a hut without ceiling fans, lights, and music?

"And cable TV," John said, now enthusiastic about the oasis.

A friend heard about the cable and brought over a twenty-seven-inch flat-screen TV. "A gift for your hut," Val said.

We had no time to mount that TV before another friend, David, saw the empty cable hookup and brought over a thirty-four-inch flat-screen TV.

Wow.

I ordered monogrammed pillows, careful with sizes and colors. "Have to be large enough to lie your head on the sofa armrest!" I insisted, having friends gauge their comfort level.

We laid a paving stone floor underneath the hut, with

wide flat walkways for wheelchair accessibility. We bought the Rolls-Royce of mosquito zappers.

We did everything possible to make the hut perfectly comfortable.

And, unwittingly, our code woes made it even more so. The placement of the hut in the middle of the yard allowed more breeze to enter it from all sides.

The first time I sat in the finished hut, I listened to the wind rustling the leaves, the pool waterfall nearby, our wind chime tinkling. I thought: I could stay here forever.

No matter how hot it is outside, it remains cool underneath the palm fronds. No matter how hard the rain pours, it remains dry. No matter how much chaos is going on inside the house or my head, the hut remains serene.

John strung small globe lights along the roof frame. At night they softly light us, brightening our lives. We never hooked up the television. Instead, we gather friends. Open some wine. Relax. Laugh.

I sit in the Chickee every day, often all day long. With the children. With friends. Mostly alone.

Wesley comes by to show me his drawings. "Look, Mom, I shaded it," he says of a precise drawing of Piglet. The shading is new. He usually draws with pens and markers, never making a mistake.

"Beautiful, Wesley," I tell him, before he wanders off.

I watch Gracie jump and run between the mango trees. She disappears into the bushes, chasing a lizard. All I can see is her white tail wagging, signaling: "Yooo-hooo! I am over here! Having a blast!"

She catches a lizard in her mouth, then drops it so it

scampers off, then catches it again. She looks puzzled—head cocked to the side, ears flopped forward—when the lizards can scamper no more.

The breeze blows. A butterfly alights. Gracie comes and lies at my feet, silently, as I write.

I rise early in the morning, a ritual change from my past life. John walks me to my favorite chair, then leaves me to my iPhone and my tapping.

If mosquitoes swarm me, I text: "Help! Spray please!"

And when nature calls, I text: "Stink pickle time. Help inside please."

John has taken to napping near me on the sofa. Covering the armrest with a big blue pillow, lying his head on it and stretching out.

"Susie—this hut was the best idea I ever had!" he said one evening, smiling.

"Seriously, it's perfect," he muttered a minute later, drifting off to sleep. "Seems like it's been here forever. Thank you."

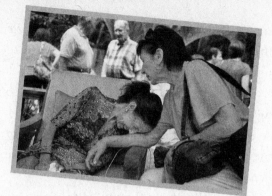

Mango Madness

I had a Mango Madness party in early June to christen the
Chickee Hut and thank the people who have helped us.
Our friends took hundreds of mangos from our trees and
cooked with them, then brought the dishes back for the party.

I invited 125. In the end, about 100 folks came. All people
who have helped me: made food, sorted photos for scrapbooks, run errands with me, pitched in to buy me an iPad,
babysat, donated money.

There was the contractor who was making our home
handicap-accessible at cost. Pat McKenna, the private detec-
tive. Droves of journalists and photographers I worked with
at the *Palm Beach Post*.

The paper's publisher came and thanked me for giving
him confidence when he first stepped into that huge role.
A former writing coach from the paper, Mary, drove from
Oklahoma. Tracey brought me a bracelet with a cross on it
and told me she was praying for me.

My neighbor—a salty sixty-something retiree—cried as he spoke to me. "I am just so sorry, Suzanne," Glenn said, his wife, Brigitte, tearing up as well.

Wesley often wanders next door to their house and asks to play, and they oblige. Wes was over so much and asked so many questions about the nude statue by their pool that Brigitte made a little modesty sarong for it.

People like that deserve a party.

John and I went all out. Borrowed tents and tables. Placed tiki torches all around the pool, waterfall, and Chickee hut. A friend hand-made decorative candles on round pieces of corkboard. We floated them in the pool.

"Your backyard is like a scene out of *Tropical Living* magazine," said one guest.

We roasted a turkey and a pig outdoors. Had margarita and pina colada slushy machines and enough booze to satiate a shipful of pirates.

At one point, some dolt pulled rather than pushed the lever on the pina colada machine. It broke, spewing coconut concoction as if from a fire hose on nearby guests.

Perfect. I LOVE memorable moments!

Our friends brought eighty-five dishes, all mango, of course. There were mango quesadillas, mango slaw, mango upside-down cake, mango and jicama salad, mango black bean salad, mango salsa and chutney, mango shrimp, mango cobbler, and much much mango more. Foodie friend Jan, of Christmas dinner fame, did a yeoman's job organizing and displaying the feast.

So there we all were in the backyard. A handful, like me, under the Chickee hut. The rest on bamboo and teak chairs, or at tables covered in tropical cloths. There were lights floating in the pool, tiki torches blazing, fresh flowers, food on plates, drinks in hand, music playing.

And it rained.

Yep, it drizzled for a good hour, just enough to dampen everything, frizz the ladies' hairdos, and hang a haze of humidity over the scene like a circus tent.

Among the guests was a man named Ron, a fifty-something former reporter we lovingly call "the cranky cousin." Ron loves to complain.

During the rain, Ron zipped over to me through the crowd and gushed: "It's wonderful, Susan. It's so wonderful. Even the rain."

The crowd migrated under the party tent and Chickee hut, chatting away in clusters. There was an occasional squeal as people who hadn't seen one another in years embraced.

Years ago at the newspaper, there was a downsizing. A passel of people took buyouts and walked out the door. The party was the largest reassembly of those folks in years. "Probably the only time they would come together like that," wrote a staffer to me afterward.

On Facebook, guests gushed it was "a magical evening!" and a "triumph by SpenWen!" Which made me smile.

At the party, I did not mingle. I did not see the banquet of food inside my home. I did not leave my chair.

When I walked, John had to hold me under my armpits, steadying me much as you would hold a toddler. I didn't want people seeing me like that.

It's called pride.

I also did not eat a bite of mango. With my weak hands, I

ate about as tidily as a two-year-old, and it's difficult for me to talk and eat without choking.

Rather, I kept a bowlful of olives next to me. Olives are (1) delicious; (2) easy to grasp, chew, and swallow; (3) mignons of high fat—more bang for the effort; and (4) salty enough to reduce the number of times hubby had to schlep me like a toddler to the bathroom.

I remember years and years ago when I flew with my infant daughter in my arms, feeling sorry for myself that I could not put my seat tray down and eat the meal. A feeling repeated scads over the years as my young children derailed many a meal: crying, pooping, spilling, fighting.

I wondered as we planned and planned the party how I would feel when I could not eat with my friends. When I could not overindulge in booze slushies, as I already struggled to walk and talk.

I wondered how I would feel watching the lovely ladies prancing in their high heels. Heels always gave me a sexy feeling, an I-am-woman-make-me-roar sensation. Loved 'em.

But after I fell and broke my clavicle, I began to give my heels away. "What size do you wear?" I'd ask someone who'd done something nice for me.

I stopped giving them away after the following epiphany: You will be able to wear them again one day in a wheelchair. Doh!

So how did I feel the night of the party about all the above? Heels? Booze? Food? Eighty-five dishes! I formerly would have waited until no one was looking and plowed my fork into every one for a taste test.

How did I feel?

I exited without a word.

It was about ten thirty, the party pulsing, the music blaring, people laughing loudly, when John helped me walk to the bathroom for the first time.

I knew then I was too tired to talk anymore, walk anymore, and asked him to help me into bed.

The stereo was right next to the bedroom. The oldie goldie by Squeeze, "Black Coffee in Bed," was playing. I fell asleep near instantly, perfectly happy.

A triumph indeed.

It wasn't till the next day in peace and quiet that I remembered that Mary, the woman who drove from Oklahoma, had handed me a small bag. "A present for later," she said.

I had set it by my chair and lost track of it.

The next morning, John asked: "Who gave you the ladybug?"

I knew it was Mary.

Now Mary and I, back in the day, were not close friends, but I respected her a great deal. And upon her retirement I sent her a card with ladybugs on it.

After my diagnosis, Mary sent me a check and mentioned that she loves ladybugs—their "blessing," as she said—and still had that card by her kitchen window.

I wrote her a thank-you note explaining that ladybugs have a special meaning to me too.

No, I don't have ladybug place mats and ladybug hand towels and ladybug salt and pepper shakers. In fact, I don't have one ladybug in my house. Just one memory of them seared in my soul.

Our nephew, Charlie, suffered for years with a rare childhood cancer called neuroblastoma. He died at age seven. He was laid to rest by his parents—John's sister Karen and her husband Bernie—in a cemetery beside a Jesuit cathedral in Pennsylvania, under a canopy of amber and gold leaves and among the graves of priests and nuns.

Two sets of grandparents, aunts, uncles, and cousins, including young children, were there. None of us knew what to say. We all stood paralyzed around the white box.

Then a swarm of ladybugs landed on it, and the small children ran up to it, laughing, trying to catch them.

I saw that as God's sign to us that He was welcoming Charlie. And in the smiles of the children, His reminder that life goes on.

I thought of that moment as I drew out Mary's gift, a small crimson-and-black enameled ladybug with rhinestone-edged wings that open to reveal a little box.

The huge party tent is now disassembled. The dishes cleaned. The coolers emptied. The slushy machines and keg returned.

The little ladybug sits on my dresser.

And life goes on.

The Journey Inward

May–June

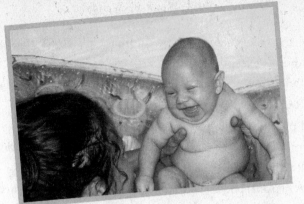

Scrapbooking

Photos. I have thousands of my children, of our travels, of our lives. Thousands.

You know those people who have all their photos squirreled away all tidy in one spot? Each labeled with the date and place?

Yeah, I am not one of those people.

I had a digital diaspora and a print disaster. I had for eons thrown pictures in shoe boxes, stowed maxed-out digital photo cards in my desk drawer, downloaded randomly to iPhoto. I was workin' and livin' so fast, I just snapped and stowed without a second glance.

In thirteen years of parenting, I had not made one photo album for any of my three children. All their firsts were buried in boxes or scattered along the information superhighway.

Oh, the shame!

After I got sick, I'd lie awake at night, thinking, Holy crap. No one but me can find the photos, much less organize and label them. No one can make photo albums for the children—except me.

Do it now.

Right now, Susan, while you still can.

I put "photo albums" on the bucket list after my diagnosis, along with the trips. A journey not out into the world, but back through my own life.

A personal photo album for each of the kids, focused on them.

A slide show of photos of my life, for anyone who wanted them.

Stories about us. Stories that turned into this book. You are holding my gift to my children. My wish that they have their mother, even after I am gone.

I started the scrapbooks in autumn, shortly after Wesley's birthday trip to the zoo. The first task? Thumb through every single picture John and I (and our friends, and even the kids) had ever taken.

You've heard it takes a village to raise children? Yeah, it took my village to make three photo albums.

My hands and arms were so weak, I could not grasp a pile of pictures or move a box. So I asked friends to help. Day after day, while Mom lay in the hospital and I planned my travels, people came to my house and thumbed through photo boxes as I watched and barked orders.

If there was one great snap of all three kids, we needed three copies. Of two kids, two copies.

My friends couldn't distinguish the boys from one another as babies. "That's Aubrey!" I'd snap, annoyed at having to say it over and over.

It was frustrating to explain repeatedly my vision of the

end product: an album for each child with every milestone. The first year, each month of miraculous growth, each birthday, each holiday, each school event, and onward.

We would make an envelope of pictures for each page, dated and labeled. I knew I would be hiring a professional scrapbooker to mount the photos. I couldn't physically do it myself, not with all the small pieces and fingerwork. So I needed organization and detail. I would give the blueprint and core material to a stranger, and she would build it.

I envisioned large, elegant leather-bound photo albums, embossed in gold, keepsakes to last my children a lifetime.

The photo sorting and labeling took months. They were social events, full of laughing, gossiping, chatting. Living while reliving.

At first, I'd linger over the adorable—the snap of roly-poly Aubrey at five months, naked in the pool, looking like a little Buddha.

Or Wesley, so chunky we couldn't button his pants.

Or Marina looking up at me with those blue eyes, smiling as she suckled at my breast.

All through Mom's illness, I lingered there. All through my trip to the Yukon, the photos stayed in their piles.

After Christmas, I realized that at the rate I was moving, I might be dead before I was done.

I ramped up the pace. Helpers arrived, and before they'd even sit down, I'd direct them to the floor. "Please spread this picture group out, and I will pick."

They would start to linger on images, asking questions.

"Let's move on," I'd say, hopefully with some veneer of politeness.

For weeks, I did this. Thumbing through memories. Printing the digital past. Blowing through ink cartridges.

"My God, this year never ends!" Nancy said as she sorted 1997, the year Marina was born.

Ack! Firstborn Marina had scads of photos, but the number dropped precipitously for each subsequent child. I started controlling for picture parity, too.

Finally, we were done. The photographs were ready to be mounted on pages, and I knew precisely what I wanted: black background, photos artfully laid out, dates noted.

I put out the call for a scrapbooker to hire. One who would treat my children's treasures as if they were her own. A lawyer friend recommended a woman named Carol.

Now here I must explain something—there is an entire industry in America of scrapbooking. There are stadium-size craft stores, Michael's being the most famous, which sell a gazillion specialty papers, borders, stamps, and scissors. They have aisle after aisle of intricate stickers of everything you can imagine, barns to bees, skyscrapers to seascapes.

E-ve-ry-thing.

Because scrapbookers pride themselves on making "theme" pages. And backgrounds. And designs.

I realized this when Carol visited with samples. My friend Missy was on hand to help me talk with Carol, since my language was slurred. I urged Missy to emphasize I wanted simple and sophisticated.

Carol was a sweet, sweet lady, about sixty, passionate about scrapbooking. And, in her mind, the more decorated a page, the better!

She showed me one theme page with a photo of a child

in a black-and-yellow bumblebee costume in the center. The background was black-and-yellow-striped paper. The photo had a scalloped border of black and yellow, and there were bumblebee stickers buzzing about. It was hard to find the child on the page.

The Fourth of July sample page was even busier. Scads of people dressed in red, white, and blue bordered in red, white, and blue with fireworks and star spangles everywhere.

I got a mild headache just looking at them. Carol and I were as different in style as Andy Warhol and Claude Monet. Me being Monet.

"The beauty is the pictures themselves," I said. "I want plain black pages where photos are the focus."

She looked horrified.

"No color?"

I harrumphed her with the following draconian edict: "You are not allowed to even GO to Michael's."

I told her I didn't wanna see one flippin' flag or bumble-bee in the books.

The color drained from her face. "But I've never done it that way," she said. "Sure I can't just use a few things?"

She pulled out an orange background paper with printed black cobwebs. "On the Halloween page?"

It was a chore to redirect Carol's design thinking. So why not shoo her away then and there?

Because I saw something in her: the way she gushed over her grandchildren, the way she viewed my children's pictures and oohed and aaahed at each one.

I knew she would handle them like the treasures they are.

A few hours later, after a pep talk from Missy, Carol

walked out the door with Wesley and Aubrey's childhoods under her arm.

Months later (I had Hungary and a cruise and Chickee hut building to oversee; Carol had surgery) she contacted me. She wanted to show me the work she had done for the boys' books and to pick up Marina's photos.

We made an appointment. Over the next few days, Steph helped me do the final prep of Marina's pictures. I realized then that I had plowed through the earlier months without feeling. I had stopped to "ooh" and "aah," but I had held my heart back.

There was my first baby before me. At two days old. Two months. Two years. Looking so sweet, so joyous. Nothing like the teen she is now, but exactly like her too.

"This process kills me," I said, slurring so badly Steph couldn't understand.

"I'm sorry. What? Calms you?"

"Never mind."

Carol came. We sat under the Chickee hut. She was nervous, wondering if finicky me would like her work. She sweated a bit.

"I called my daughter this morning and asked her to wish me luck!" Carol told me, with a worried chuckle.

It's odd how a ninety-five-pound disabled woman can be so intimidating.

But I know why: Carol didn't want to let me down.

Carol pulled dozens of completed pages from her roller bag. She had neatly stowed my original photo envelope with each page. I could see the handwriting of the various friends who helped assemble, which delighted me.

The pages had a black background, with a drop of color. Carol had sparingly bordered each photo in a color that complemented the subject, but did not overpower it. She had neatly labeled in finely cut letters.

The pages were gorgeous. "I love them," I said.

Carol sighed. "I am so relieved."

I shall linger for the rest of my days over the finished books, the job done, no longer plowing through.

I shall relive my children's childhoods, as I hope they will one day. I hope they will see in front of them what beautiful people they are.

And how much their mother loved them.

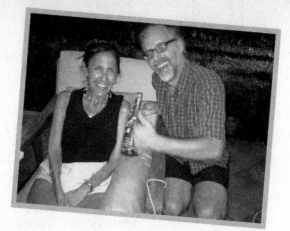

Stink Pickle

Monday, June 11, two days after the Mango Madness party, was the day I finally had to ask my husband to wipe me.

And the day someone offered to publish my book.

Life is funny like that. Perfect like that.

I had passed a stink pickle, just like always, when I realized I could no longer reach around and wipe with torpedo accuracy. My right arm, the last one working, was impossible to control at that angle. My hand was too furled to spread out my paper squares.

"John! Help!"

Poor John. We'd known this day would come and discussed stink pickle protocol ahead of time. "As long as I don't have to stare at 'em, I'll be fine," John said. "Please flush before you call me in."

"Roger."

So I flushed, and he came in.

I crouched, and he leaned me forward, nearly toppling me on my head.

"Sorry," he eked out, holding his breath.

He wiped and wiped and wiped. I finally had to snap: "That's enough! It's my ass. I know!"

Now, we could have despaired at that moment. But I had forsworn despair. And we had far better things to do. Namely, check my e-mail.

I had been writing ever since my diagnosis. Actually, I had been writing all my life, but I'd been writing about myself since the diagnosis: my triumphs, my falls, my attempt to live with joy and die with joy. I'd been writing the story of my life, as seen through one great year.

On Christmas Day, the *Palm Beach Post* had published my article on my Yukon trip with Nancy. In May, they published an article on my trip with John to Hungary. I received some of the best feedback of my career. People wrote to cheer me on. Someone said they hadn't cried in seventeen years, but they cried when they read about my journey.

Poor John. Women gushed over his line from the Hungary article: "It's not a burden. The least I can do for you is everything."

"But it's true," he said sadly.

Then, as things do, the hubbub died down. I went back to Chickee huts and friends, planning trips and laughing about Marina's teenage drama.

Then an old colleague, Charles Passy, called. He liked my articles and wanted to mention them in his *Wall Street Journal* blog. It wasn't a printed article, just a long blog entry on the paper's website.

I asked Charles to please include that I hoped to publish the book I was writing.

The next day an agent called me. He had heard about the blog from a friend, who heard about it from another friend . . . you get the picture.

An hour later, I was on a call with the agent. We chatted. I liked him. 'Nuff said.

Peter, ever the agent, started explaining book deals. 'Nuff said, Peter! 'Nuff said.

"I can barely talk," I told him. "I can barely walk. I don't care about the details. You're hired. Let's get 'er done."

And next thing ya know, I was on conference calls with producers from ABC and Disney, and I had a New York City lawyer, former general counsel of Simon & Schuster.

Stephanie stood by for the calls, helping clarify my slurred speech. "Drop lotsa F-bombs when ya talk for me so they know I might not be Disney material," I told her beforehand.

Soon an offer came from a major publishing house. I was thrilled. Peter wanted to try for more.

"Go for it!" I said.

This was Friday. I had a mango party to prepare for the next day. I had a memory to make.

"This is going nuclear!" Peter wrote me on Monday morning as I sat on the toilet. "A BIG offer is coming."

After my stink pickle, I ran to my phone. Okay, okay, John put his hands under my armpits and walked me slowly, step by step, back to the Chickee hut, pausing for a long moment at that pesky step that led down from our pool. But in my mind, I ran.

No messages.

"What will come will come," I told myself. "What is meant to be is meant to be."

I put my iPhone down. I sat on the steps of my pool with Stephanie. Spent time with Wesley. Laid in the guest bed to rest, ate a few bites—all I could chew—and watched *Law & Order*.

When I returned to my phone, there were a host of missed calls from New York and e-mails with the subject line: "Big offer!!! Where are you??"

"Light me a cigarette!" I said to Yvette, my helper.

Breathe.

I dialed Peter.

"Are you sitting down?" he asked.

I was so distracted, I didn't even think of the snappy comeback: "Yes, dear. I can't stand up."

He told me the offer. It was BIG. Not quite as big as later reported in the newspapers (even my beloved *Palm Beach Post*), but big enough to send my kids to college. For John to quit his job, if he wanted, and go back to school to become a physician's assistant. For me to leave my family well off.

"I think we should go with it," Peter said.

"I promise to make you proud," I told him. "I am confident I can do this. I will write until the day I die."

I saw the struggle on John's face when I told him the news. I knew what he was thinking. I had heard him say it a hundred times, with his words and eyes. "I know you want me to be happy. I know you need me to be happy. But I'm just so sad."

He was conflicted. My illness had led to the book. It was my life for financial freedom. A terrible trade.

"I just want you to be well."

"I know."

"I'd rather have you than the money."

"But it doesn't work that way," I said. "This is the best possible outcome of the worst possible scenario. It is my gift to you."

That night, I lay beside my husband and marveled anew at the yin and yang of everything. It wasn't a trade. It was life.

A day begun in indignity had ended in the extraordinary. Perfect.

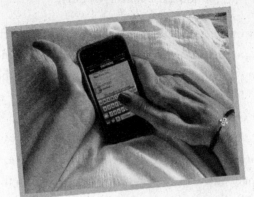

My Triathlon

I started writing full-time the next day.

I realized immediately that, as with the scrapbooks, my pace had been too slow. I had spent my time wandering through my life, in and out of happy moments, jotting them down casually. I had maybe 10 percent of a book complete—and only a few months of coordination left.

I took a deep breath.

I had a triathlon to run.

But I wasn't worried.

I had been training for this most of my adult life. Banging out stories from the courtrooms of Palm Beach County, my front-row seat for the flotsam and jetsam of humanity.

Stories, too often, about teenage thugs sentenced to life, some without a parent in sight. About victims mowed down by drunk drivers, their families weeping so hard the courtroom benches shook. About husbands hiring hit men to whack wives, and vice versa.

Sometimes the crimes were so senseless, they made me angry. Sometimes the criminals so neglected I found myself wondering if society was to blame. Sometimes the details so brutal, I went home each night and hugged my children, thanking God we were all right.

But occasionally, the stories went the other way. I pro-filed a state supreme court justice, Barbara Pariente, who got breast cancer and kept working, appearing bald on the bench.

I wrote a long piece on a homeless woman, Angel Gloria Gonzalez, who taught herself the law, represented herself in a federal complaint, and got her eviction overturned on the basis of racial discrimination.

"This never happens," I told her straight up. "You are unique."

My proudest moment as a journalist, though, was the time I tracked down four killers and crossed our top prosecutor to tell a story nobody involved wanted told.

It started with a plot to murder a beautiful blonde named Heather Grossman. Her ex-husband, Ron Samuels, was a megalomaniac businessman who always got what he wanted. And he didn't want Heather alive, not after she got custody of the kids.

It wasn't that Ron didn't love his three young children, Ron's new wife later testified. It's that he hated paying child support.

So Ron turned to a crack-addicted friend, who turned to a crack dealer, who hired two crack addicts to "whack the wife." On October 14, 1997, one of them—Roger Runyon—loaded a high-powered rifle and fired at the base of Heather's skull as she and her new husband sat at a stoplight.

Heather survived, a quadriplegic.

Ron Samuels was eventually arrested and tried for attempted murder. In October 2006, he was convicted and sentenced to life. The other four conspirators walked free. They had been given immunity in exchange for their testimony.

I sat near Heather Grossman in the courtroom for weeks. I saw her pushed down the aisle in her wheelchair day after day, her head permanently slumped on its rest. I watched tears roll sideways into her ear and listened to the machine breathing for her, *sh-sh-sh-shewww*, one mechanical puff after another.

I will know that feeling soon.

But my disease will render me so. Heather Grossman was shot. Four men plotted. One put a bullet in her brain.

Did they have to go free?

The top prosecutor's flak told me, "There's no story here, Susan." And, "None of the networks covered it." And it will only "piss off" the top man.

As a journalist, you know you are onto something good when people say stuff like that.

So I researched the case and discovered there had been evidence to charge and prosecute the men. I discovered that the testimony of Roger Runyon, the shooter, did not directly implicate Ron Samuels. Yet he had been given immunity in advance and walked free.

I tracked down the would-be killers.

To a life insurance agency in Hollywood, Florida, where one of the conspirators told me the immunity deal was "the best thing I ever did." To an office in Deerfield Beach. To a flop house in Carol City, north of Miami.

I flew to Indianapolis and drove to the small town in Indiana where the shooter, Roger Runyon, lived. His house was on a rural highway at the edge of a cornfield.

I stood at his front door, attempting to interview him. A wild turkey in his yard began chasing me. I heard him inside, but he wouldn't answer the door.

I talked to the local police chief and Runyon's parole officer. He was on probation for traffic violations. Neither knew he had once shot to kill in Florida.

It felt important to write that story, so that readers would understand the dynamics behind our criminal system. It felt important to let them know how complex justice can be— and how far-reaching the ramifications.

But it felt personal too.

I love that story because I loved Heather Grossman. She inspired me with her will to live after the crippling shot. With her tenacity raising her children. With how beautiful and strong she seemed in her wheelchair, even with her body lost.

She couldn't breathe on her own. She couldn't live on her own. But she competed in Mrs. Wheelchair America. I mean, the clams on this girl.

Write about strength, I told myself, as I sat in my Chickee hut. Don't write about your disease. Write about joy.

I was stunned, a few months ago, by a documentary about Heather's case. Years after the shooting, Heather saw the emergency room surgeon who had operated on her. The doctor told her she had begged him not to save her life.

Heather had not remembered. She wept as she recounted it more than decade later, her children nearly adults. "I am so glad the doctor didn't listen to me!" she cried.

Be honest, I told myself.

We can despair. Like Heather Grossman. Like me. It's what we summon after the tragedy—the tenacity—that matters.

By June, I had lost the ability to use my iPad. The keyboard was too big, and it tired my right hand to move it back and forth.

I decided to write the book using the "notes" function on my iPhone instead. John or Stephanie, or even Aubrey or Marina if they were around, would slide the phone into my useless left hand, where by serendipity my curled fingers formed a perfect holder. I would type each letter with my right thumb—tap! tap!—the only digit I could control.

I added "Thank God for Technology" as my e-mail tagline, for I realized that five years ago, before the touchscreen typing pad, this book would have been impossible for me.

I tapped and tapped away.

I rose early, willing myself to finish a chapter every day. I wrote through the weekends. I wrote when I was traveling with my loved ones. At one point, knowing how weak I was becoming, I committed to write forty chapters in one month (some were cut or combined by my editor). I accomplished it, though I took two major trips during that time.

Such is the power of desire.

When people came over, I asked them to take the phone from my hand (since I could not hand it to them) and read the latest section out loud (since I could no longer read aloud). On the iPhone, I could see only twenty or thirty words at a time. I wanted to hear the cadence and flow.

I had my favorite sections read over and over to me by different visitors. I could not hug them. I did not go out for meals with them or to the beach. I could not walk the yard or hold a conversation for more than a few minutes.

These sections, read in the cool shade of the Chickee hut, were my conversations. I was speaking to my family and friends with my written words, and I was reliving the moments.

Meeting John. My children's births. The peace I embraced inside.

Sometimes a word or turn of phrase made me smile.

Sometimes I would smile with anticipation, knowing a favorite line was coming soon.

(Like Soulla, when I asked about the man in the photo: "That's your grandmother!")

When I wrote with others present, it frustrated me. Like when I would watch Nancy typing away quickly on her phone, then think about my own slow pace—an effort to push each letter.

But writing this book was not work. Like each journey I took during the year, it brought me joy. It kept me alive.

Like every good thing in my life, I didn't want it to end.

When I typed the last letter of the first draft in mid-September, three months after beginning in earnest, I couldn't believe what I had accomplished.

I felt as if I'd pulled myself up a mountain with nine fingers tied behind my back.

I let the moment linger, the thrill of a triathlon completed.

I looked at John, who was sitting across from me in the

Chickee hut. I expected to smile. To beam with the dream fulfilled.

I cried.

And formed the words as best I could: "What will I do now?"

Letting Go

May–June

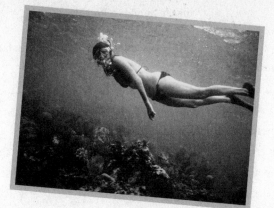

Swimming

Today, June 21, is the summer solstice. Not today in the book. I mean that I am sitting in my Chickee hut right now, writing this sentence with one finger on the longest day of sunlight of the year. One of my favorite days.

I am a sun baby, born and raised in Florida, where sun chaperones our lives. I brown up like a coffee bean. A Greek gift (thank you, Panos), so I have always enjoyed full sun.

Take me to a restaurant, and I'll elect the sunny seat. Take me camping on nearby Peanut Island, and I will while away the entire day standing in waist-deep crystal water, hand-feeding the fish or snorkeling the cove, searching for manatees.

Did you know small fish will eat dog biscuits straight from your hand?

I was a scuba diver years ago, and one of the highlights for me was looking to the surface of the ocean from sixty feet underneath, seeing the sun's rays shooting silver through the water. At that depth, on a sunny day, the ocean's surface looks like mercury.

I used to float near the shore as the waves rolled in, churning up shells. If you are still and listen underwater, you can hear them tinkling. Delight.

My friend and I used to stand on one another's shoulders in the water and front-flip off. I once kneed myself in the eye doing this, leaving a shiner.

Yes, I could sun and swim all day, every day, my solar chaperone following my every move, toasting my shoulders and back. No sunscreen.

"I musta been a reptile in another life," I used to say as I baked.

I fell for John, a tan collegiate swimmer, in his Speedo. Behind my dark Ray-Bans, I tracked his fluid freestyle strokes. His muscular arms—his "guns," as he jokingly calls them—zipped him through the water with nary a splash.

(A typical John crack: "I need to go to the vet." "Why?" Flexes his arms. "Because these pythons are sick.")

I too was a competitive swimmer. Not a great one. A decent one. So John and I would work out in the pool.

"Okay, sprints," he'd order.

I'd buzz fast as I could across the pool, convinced I was windmilling my arms faster than Janet Evans, the tiny woman who Roto-Rootered her way to umpteen gold medals in the late 1980s and early '90s. And John would say: "No. Let's sprint."

"I am."

"Really?"

I think of that now as I stare at our backyard pool on this

sunny summer solstice. Recently, some friends and I were hanging out around that pool, drinking a beer, when I asked to go in. Two people—it now takes two people, if they aren't experienced like John and Steph—helped me onto the pool steps. I sat there, half submerged, drinking my beer through a straw.

My back was to the group, so I tried to float onto my stomach and face them.

As I turned, my head dipped and I inhaled water. Like a child learning to swim, I felt the burn up my nostrils. I was shocked. I opened my mouth and inhaled more.

Didn't have the strength to lift my head.

The folks heard me sputtering. Four hands grabbed me, pulled me up.

"I'm okay," I said.

I returned to sitting on the step with my back to them. I realized I could probably no longer swim.

This was not something I announced, trying not to trigger the cascade of I'm-sorrys. I struggled with that fact alone.

Since then, I have not asked anyone to get in the pool with me to test my hypothesis. Truth is, I don't want to know. If it's gone, it's gone. Nothing I can do. Slipped away like a charm off a necklace.

So how shall I handle it? Pine away for something I can no longer do? Something I adored?

No.

For that is the path to the loony bin. To want something you can never have.

"I am the master of my mind. I have a choice about how to feel," I tell myself all the time.

I have practiced this again and again over the last few years: the art of letting go.

I used to be a regular in the hundred-degree room at a local Bikram yoga studio. The heat of the room helped expand not only my muscles but my mind as well.

Yoga was my refuge from the Chinese fire drill of modern life. I could walk into a Bikram class hoarding angst, and exit with my muscles stretched and my mind swept clean by ninety minutes of exertion so intense I didn't have the energy to worry about a thing.

When I realized I could no longer grip with my left hand, I refused to accept my loss. I put on a weightlifting glove and kept going to yoga. Then I noticed the fingers of my left hand would no longer lie neatly side by side.

When I lifted my hand above my head, it looked like a star atop a Christmas tree.

I did yoga for my neurologist, right in his office. Lifted my left leg up, up, up behind me, gripping my ankle in a standing bow, one of Bikram's most difficult positions. Nailed it. Proof, I insisted, that I didn't have ALS.

I lost yoga six months later, with sadness.

A year after that, I casually mentioned to John, "Did you know I can't jump anymore?" as if it were an observation about a recent shopping trip.

When our neighbor told me she no longer wanted me to drive with her children in the car, I fumed. I told John, still angry hours later, and he said, "Susan, I don't feel that good about our kids riding with you either."

Now that hurt.

Two months later, driving my beloved BMW, I pulled

over to the side of the road and told Stephanie, without tears or drama, "I don't think I should drive anymore. I'm having trouble steering."

Acceptance.

Control.

Remember child killer Nathaniel Brazill? He was a seventh-grader when he shot his teacher at the classroom door in 2000. The incident took place a few miles from my house. I was the first reporter to view the surveillance tape, one of the biggest scoops of my career.

A decade later, I interviewed Brazill in prison. "Prison's not a bad place," he told me. "It doesn't really seem like punishment."

I wrote the story for the *Palm Beach Post*, and people were disgusted. They called his attitude "evidence" that he was a cold-blooded criminal.

I called his attitude "survival." Nathaniel Brazill had to reinvent his environs to survive. Prison is not a bad place, he convinced himself.

And not swimming, after a lifetime of doing so, doesn't have to be so bad either.

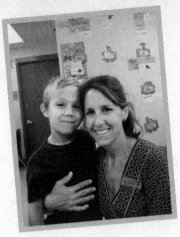

Aubrey's Birthday

June 18, 2012, five days ago, was my son's birthday. A day to stop. To contemplate and be proud. My Aubrey was turning eleven years old.

What a memory, the day he was born! I was fully preggers. Overdue, in fact. My due date was June 14, but I asked the doctor to wait on the C-section. I wanted June 21, the summer solstice. I envisioned his birthday parties stretching into the eve on the longest day, the sunlight lifting him.

On June 18, I reported all day from the courthouse. I was lying down afterward, resting, when three-year-old Marina started jumping on the bed.

"Stop!" barked John. "You may hurt Mommy."

I got up, went to the bathroom to pee, and felt a whoosh of water. John and I stood over the toilet examining the liquid. Yes, staring into the toilet bowl, trying to divine our future.

"You think your water broke?" he asked.

"No, it can't be."

I had such a plan for how I wanted my baby born, I reinvented what was happening. No, the liquid running down my leg was obviously incontinence. And the viscous spots in the toilet water were, oh, something else.

I laid back down, still dreaming of my summer solstice baby.

Then I had a contraction.

Marina had been born by C-section, after that school bus ride in Bogota. I'd had no labor, no experience with this vise grip on my abdomen.

If there is one thing in the world that will fast-forward you right into reality, it is said vise grip. And the horrific thought of a breech birth, a foot emerging and the doc tugging out the tangled little soul.

In no time, we were on our way to the hospital.

Now, John and I had been disagreeing for months over names. John wanted . . . okay, I can't remember what John wanted, but he was not keen on the name Aubrey.

"It sounds like a girl's name," John kept saying. "People will think he's Audrey."

After a while, I stopped talking of it. But I never let the name go. It was important to me.

You see, Aubrey was an older cousin of mine: Aubrey Motz IV, to be exact. That Aubrey was a severe hemophiliac. His blood would not clot properly. Bump him too hard, and he would bleed internally.

He once went for a boat ride with us and ended up hospitalized with a bleed on his brain. He is the reason, I think, my parents decided not to bear kids of their own.

Aubrey Motz used blood products all his life to help his body clot its blood. Sometime in the early 1990s, before blood was vetted for HIV, he received an infected batch. He died of AIDS in 1999. He was thirty-nine years old.

Aubrey was my favorite cousin. He was intelligent, funny, kind, and—the juggernaut for me—he never complained. He had not an angry bone in his frail body.

Life served him a double whammy, first a chronic illness, then a fatal one. Yet Aubrey lived with joy and no self-pity. He went to college, he traveled, he married. He lived.

After he died, I thought of him often. I still do. I try every day to emulate him. I didn't want four generations of his name to die with him. I wanted to honor his memory.

So I waited until I was on the operating table, ready to be sliced open. After nearly vomiting—an effect of the anesthesia—I brought up the name again.

"Please, let's name him Aubrey."

What could John say at that moment but yes?

In exchange, John got to name our third child. He chose Atticus, after Atticus Finch in *To Kill a Mockingbird*, his favorite book. We've never called Wesley by his first name.

On my first outing with baby Aubrey to the library, I heard a mother calling, "Aubrey!" and saw her daughter toddle over. Ruh-roh!

Then Aubrey's first birthday cake came back from the bakery with big frosted letters: "Happy Birthday, Audrey!"

Yet I am so glad I named my boy Aubrey, for there is value in a family name. The continuity. The memories. I tell my Aubrey about his namesake. I note how he never complained, because truth be told, my Aubrey's chief negative trait—and by Jove, we all have 'em—is, he's a complainer.

Just the other day, when I told him he wouldn't get his BIG birthday present until 7:00 p.m., the exact hour he was born, he rolled his eyes. "Oh, gosh!" he said. "I am not even eleven yet."

Of my three children, Aubrey is the one I worry for the most.

His brother Wesley, insulated by Asperger's, doesn't crave affection and remains blissfully unaware of my impending death. Wes's chief concern is that HE be the one to push my wheelchair when we go out.

His sister, Marina, has the ginormous distraction of boys and friends and fashion and high school.

And then there's my Aubrey. The middle one. Squashed between his special-needs brother and a teenage sister who currently regards him as a sixty-five-pound pain in the ass. My most sensitive and sentient child.

At his parent-teacher conference this year, his teacher told me: "Aubrey's an old soul." Which broke my heart. For old souls are wiser souls. Wise to what's going on around them.

Indeed, Aubrey was the first (and so far only) of my children to ask directly about my condition.

Aubrey was the first to offer to help me without prompting. When my walking began to falter, he would step beside me so I could put my hand on his neck for balance.

He checks on me often, popping his head out our back door, hollering to me parked out in the Chickee hut writing, "You okay, Mom?"

Perhaps this is his old soul. Or perhaps it is the fact he's seen me in some pretty pitiful states.

Like the time, a few weeks after I got back from the Yukon, I went to pick him up from school. A new opportunity I treasured since leaving work. I was early that day, so I went inside to use the bathroom. I was walking down a little-used hallway when I slipped and fell, ker-plunk, flat on my back.

I wriggled like a beetle, unable to get up. Wondering what to do.

Then Aubrey and another boy happened to walk by.

"Mom!" he said, running to my side, but not before glancing at the other boy to see if he was watching.

For the first time, I felt my condition embarrassed my son.

The other boy walked off, and Aubrey started trying to hoist me up, grabbing me under the armpits, tugging me toward my feet.

"Whoa, Nellie! Slow down," I said. "Let me catch my breath."

His hazel eyes were flung wide. "Don't worry," I said. "I am fine. Ready?"

He tried again and nearly toppled over. I laughed, so he started too.

"Okay. Help me turn over on all fours and crawl to the door. I can grab the door handle."

When I reached the door, I directed him to grab the top of the back of my pants and pull. "It's okay. Give me a big wedgie!"

It worked. I got up. I went to the bathroom and walked out of school with my son by my side, my arm draped around his neck for balance.

A few days later, as I exited school with Aubrey, some woman walked up to me and blurted out, "What happened to you?"

If Aubrey had been not been standing there, I would have replied, "What happened to your face?"

Because it hurt. How must I look, I wondered, if that woman spoke to me like that?

Soon after, I sat down and wrote an e-mail to Aubrey's and Wesley's teachers. I knew they had seen me stumble and slur. I didn't want them to misunderstand. I told them I didn't have a drinking problem. I had a disease.

Then I stopped picking my kids up from school. Dad took over. One more favor asked. One more thing I couldn't do.

One thing I never thought I'd miss so much.

Now, six months later, I worried I was disappointing Aubrey again.

I have always made a big to-do about birthdays. I buy two or three colors of streamers, and the night before John and I string them from the center chandelier to all corners of our Florida room—the tropical equivalent of a den. The child awakes to a canopy of color.

This year, I could no longer zip myself over to Party City. And I forgot to remind John.

Aubrey awoke to the same old house.

Then there was the cake. I always bought special cakes, covered in silky fondant or glazed in ganache. Or made my own, not nearly as fancy, but not for lack of effort.

Last year, I got out my Wilton icing tips and icing bags and piped a fancy trim on a homemade cake.

Aubrey's party was at a local water park in full Florida sun. By lunchtime, the piping was dripping off the cake like sweat. Aubrey and the gaggle of ten-year-olds ended up ravaging it with spoons.

This year, I couldn't manage a cake. So Steph stepped in and took Aubrey to the grocery store. He chose a Smurf cake. Yes, Smurfs. A bastion of blue icing. Stephanie made him a steak dinner as I napped with Gracie.

In the evening, we gathered for cake and presents. A few days before, I had upgraded to another iPhone and wrapped up my old one for Aubrey. Marina had gotten a new phone for her eleventh birthday, some cheapo model. I reasoned old was okay, since Aubrey was getting a much nicer phone than his sister had.

We sang "Happy Birthday" and ate blue cake, the liter of dye leaving everyone looking cyanotic with blue lips.

Aubrey opened the phone, in its original packing box. He loved it. Immediately began plugging in everyone's numbers and texting away.

Hmmm. Still no complaints? Perhaps I was the only one who missed traditions so.

About an hour later, Aubrey came to me in the Chickee hut. "Look, there's a scratch. Is this your old phone?"

"Yes."

"Marina didn't get a used phone!"

"Marina didn't get an iPhone. Quit complaining."

He sauntered off into the house and texted me: "Thank you."

The next day, while at a friend's house, he texted me: "Are you ok?"

"Yes," I replied.

Then he texted me symbols. "Eye-heart-u."

"Eye-heart-u too my son."

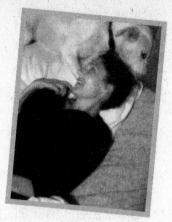

Helping Hands

Sweet Gracie, our gold-eyed girl.

While my children, thankfully, went on with their normal lives, my dog knew something was wrong with me. She grew more and more antsy through my long period of nesting that spring, until she finally ate the strap off my bikini top. She had chewed shoes before (preferring the supple Italian leather ones), but not clothing.

I used to place my breast-milk-stained shirt in the crib with my babies. The scent seemed to comfort them. I wondered if Gracie chewing my clothing might be the same thing.

No bother. I did not miss the bathing suit.

I chose to appreciate the gesture. For Gracie, and her antics, comforted me. She was often my sole companion in the Chickee hut, usually curled at my feet. Or chasing lizards and jumping at squirrels, which was just as nice.

When I napped in the afternoon, she hopped on the bed and licked my face. I know. Gross. But I loved it.

Sometimes she curled around my head on the pillow, her long tongue slinking down the sides of my face. More often, she plopped down atop my chest for a full frontal lick-fest.

Thwack! Thwack! pounded her tail on the mattress as she licked, no end in sight, her sixty pounds making it hard for me to breathe.

"Help!" I'd called out, and as I opened my mouth, in darted her tongue.

Eeeeewwwww! Gross! Even I have standards.

Once, in her excitement, Gracie moved up for a better lick and put her paw on my throat. Now I really couldn't breathe, and I was too weak to push her off.

"Help!" I squeaked. "Help!"

Aubrey tottered in. "Gracie! You killin' Mommy?" he said, tugging her off me by her collar.

He exited the room to return to his regularly scheduled activity. Gracie hopped right back on the bed.

"Off! Off!" I told her, before giving up and letting the dog lie.

Early each evening, usually before bedtime for the children, John walks me step by step to our bedroom.

He takes off my clothing piece by piece.

He puts me on the toilet.

Brushes my teeth.

Lays me in the bed.

"Is there anything else you need?"

"Just bring in Gracie," I tell him.

She hops on the bed with me. She curls around the pillow and slinks her tongue across my face. I think of Wesley, and how she does the same for him. She puts us both to sleep.

Once, in the middle of the night, I awoke alone in the guest room at the north end of our house, far away from the other bedrooms.

I had to use the bathroom, but needed help to get out of bed. I called out in the darkness: "Hello! Hello!"

No response.

I waited for our noisy air conditioner to cycle off and tried again. "Hello! Hello!" I called out, my weak voice rising with the pressure in my bladder.

No response. No one awoke.

"Hello! Hello! Help! Help!"

In came Gracie, probably from Wesley's bed. She looked at me, head cocked quizzically. Then began barking loudly, right outside Marina's bedroom door.

Marina awoke and got John to help me.

"Just like Lassie!" I said on the toilet.

She started following me, underfoot at the most inopportune moments, like when John helped me to the bathroom.

"Hurry! Hurry!" I said, trying to avoid an accident.

And there was Gracie, right in the way, scampering into the tiny bathroom alongside the two of us.

"Gracie! Out!" John hollered, annoyed.

On various occasions, our sixty-pound girl has nearly knocked me over, jumping on me or sideswiping me while I tried to stand.

"We should get rid of the dog," John said one day in anger.

"Over my dead body," I replied.

Gracie goes nuts when the kids jump in the pool, barking,

leaping into trees, tugging off the bark. We had to wrap some trunks in chicken wire.

But Gracie never ever jumps in the pool—except once.

John was giving Aubrey a whale ride, our name for Aubrey clinging to his back while John swims deep underwater. The two stayed under the water, gliding along the bottom, an unusually long time. Gracie musta thought they were drowning.

She jumped in and swam toward them.

Then John and Aubrey surfaced, and Gracie climbed right out.

Lassie!

Poor John. Parent. Caregiver. Dog walker. Tired soul. Each morn, he wipes paw prints off our upholstery, muttering about the damn dog.

I've heard of husbands emotionally abandoning their sick wives. Not John. I think he feels my pain as much as I do, my frustration at all the little things I cannot do. Things like pulling myself up from a toilet or lifting my own feet.

Now John has to do them for me.

He has help. Believe me, when you can't put on your own shoes, you aren't shy about asking for assistance. My friend Jane Smith, who planned my retirement party from the *Post* and bought my iPad, set up an entire schedule of helpers on WhatFriendsDo.com.

But sometimes, like with Gracie, that help made it harder on John. There were friends in and out of the house all day— running errands, bringing meals—but I had trouble communicating my wishes, or even thanking them.

I couldn't get out of my chair, for one thing. Fortunately,

we have an open-door policy. We've always been one of those houses where the door is unlocked all day and neighborhood kids, relatives, and do-gooders just walk right in.

Which was a blessing, since I was so often out in my backyard Chickee. And I couldn't answer the door, even if I wanted to. Couldn't turn the knob. Couldn't really be social, even when people sat with me. Too hard with my lazy tongue. Too tiring.

I sent John out to buy a bunch of marsala cooking wine. I wanted to give my favorite recipe—Shrimp Onassis, which called for marsala—to each person who cooked for us.

"Here is the secret ingredient, marsala, which transforms the recipe. Just as your kindness has transformed this day for me," I had John write in the thank-you notes.

It was hard on him. He was coming home from work and having to chase kids, greet edible gift–bringers (many of whom he'd never met), and hand them wine, when half the time he couldn't locate it or remember what to write.

All while I was texting him I had to pee, so he needed to walk me to the bathroom . . . right now.

And Wesley, God love him, but he was TALKING LIKE THIS THE WHOLE TIME, and not having a conversation, just talking round and round about whatever was on his mind.

"Can I take a picture of Gracie? Do you like lizards? Did you see the book I drew? It's the ugly duckling. See, he's crying. But over here, his mom found him, and he's happy now."

Thank goodness for Yvette, our amazing housekeeper. Wesley loved Yvette. They could talk Piglet and *Lilo & Stitch* for hours. I think Wesley watched that movie ten times in a row.

Actually, it wasn't the movie. It was the ad for the movie on the on-demand channel. He watched the ad a hundred times, until Stephanie rented the movie for him one night.

Delight.

Meanwhile, the food piled up. Everyone was so generous, bringing enough for eight. But Marina was often away with friends. Aubrey and Wesley were picky boys. And my appetite was down to half of what it once was, maybe less.

That left John. The man can eat, but not for seven and a half.

"Tell them thank you, but we're fine for now," John told me, when we discussed the frequent food drops.

"You say it," I grumped. "I can barely talk."

The frustration culminated in a meltdown. Of course I have them. My mind is untouched by ALS. I get furious sometimes.

Like when we didn't have the proper wine bags to put the damn gift wines in.

John stopped chasing Gracie at that one and looked at me. "Did you miss your medication?"

At my first appointment with the neurologist, I had asked for an antidepressant. I was prescribed 10 mg of Lexapro a day, the smallest amount. After my diagnosis, the doctor doubled the dosage to 20 mg. We called it my "happy pill."

"Yes," I said, realizing what had happened.

Like Road Runner, John darted to the medicine cabinet.

He placed the chalky pill toward the back of my tongue. As usual, it stuck and dissolved there, gagging me. No muscle to push it down.

Bitter, then bitter again, swooshing back into my mouth.

I gestured to John to bring the water cup close. Real close, where I could put my lips around the straw, no hands. The only way I could drink.

The only way to swallow the bitter pill that helps make me happy.

Recently I switched to liquid Lexapro, no longer able to swallow a pill. It's no less bitter, but I would gargle garlic if it helped me feel better.

Is there a stigma to admitting depression? To admitting that I have moments of anger and despair? If so, I choose to ignore it, because my mind is healthy.

It is like running a marathon. Even trained, the marathon is grueling. But you can complete it.

Even on antidepressants, ALS is devastating. But I can complete it.

For the depression comes less frequently now. Since my diagnosis. Since acceptance. It swoops in like a butterfly, landing silently as they do on the bushes near the Chickee hut. I watch it flutter, admiring the complexity. I feel its weight for a moment, then it's gone.

That kind of sadness has a beauty. It lets me know I am alive.

And that I still care.

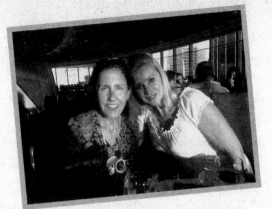

Hospice

The months visiting my mother in the hospital never left me. The nights I spent lying awake in her room, looking, thinking, feeling. Watching as the nurses checked medication and vitals. Listening to the whirring of the IV drips, their alarms *BB-RRRing*-ing in the night. Smelling the feeding-tube liquid, a milky-looking substance with a scent all its own.

And it ain't like pot roast.

Dad visited three or four times a day. He endured the brunt of Mom's frustration and confusion. Her fear. At one juncture, Mom just shot birds at Dad, who had shown nothing but absolute care for her. She would not even watch TV.

Dad was so strained, I wondered when he would snap. Then he had to tackle end-of-life issues, uncertain what Mom would want.

Those images, those moments, those *smells*, will stay with me forever. In the following months, I lived them over and over again. This was not the butterfly of depression, swooping down to my shoulder and then flying away. This was not self-pity.

What I saw in the hospital gave me a clear-eyed view of myself. It made me vow not to put my loved ones through the same. I did not want John to agonize over whether to cease medical intervention. I would not run my family into the ground with endless hospital stays.

If I had to die, I decided, I would die as gracefully as possible.

I talked and talked with John, making sure he understood my wishes. Chief among them that I never languish in a hospital.

Unlike my mother's illness, there was no hope of recovery from ALS.

I had the necessary legal documents drawn up. No hospital. No ventilator. No artificial feeding. No measures to prolong life when at the hairy edge of death.

Easier for me.

Easier for my family.

Not giving up, but accepting.

And who knew better how to honor that spirit than hospice? Hospice services offer palliative care. They comfort the dying, instead of treating them.

"Sign me up!" I told John.

No, I'll sign myself up while I still can, I thought. Better they shall hear my wishes in my own words, before I can talk no more.

I contacted Hospice of Palm Beach County. The hospice intake nurse came to our house. A friend took our children to the movies. Stephanie and her husband Don joined John and me. We opened a bottle of red wine.

"Am I doing the right thing?" I asked Steph and Don.

They are both respiratory therapists and have worked in hospitals. Don's job was helping manage gravely ill people on life-support ventilators. He often saw families maintaining a loved one after realistic hope of recovery was gone.

"Absolutely," Don told me. "You are doing the right thing."

Stephanie had seen patients passing into death in the hospital. "The last place anyone should die," she said.

About ten times in her career she had remained with patients, holding their hands while they died, because no one else was doing so. "I just never want anyone alone at that time," she said.

The hospice worker was a sunny lady with a Caribbean accent. I cannot remember her name, but liked her very much. She was matter-of-fact about death, and not one bit maudlin.

I remember laughing as we kept offering her wine. We opened a second bottle. "No, thank you," she said. "But I'm surely havin' a taste when I get home!"

How did I feel?

Good. Like I was giving a gift to my family. Sad, of course. But good.

For hours the hospice nurse stayed (we kept sidetracking her with stories), completing paperwork. Mounds of paperwork. Fifteen copies of everything, each needing to be signed. She asked me question after question about my condition.

I remember one about my loss of weight.

I explained I had little appetite. Yes, I could swallow. But yes, the difficulty of having others prepare food and feed me diminished my desire. I usually ate just once daily.

"It's natural," she said. "I tell my families all the time, the dying don't eat as much. Their body doesn't need it."

Ah! That explains it. So natural.

I was emphatic that I wanted no hospital stay.

Sometimes, she explained, it was unavoidable to manage a condition causing great pain and discomfort. She asked in that scenario where I would like to be taken.

I had seen the hospice wing at my mother's hospital, its dimly lit hallways painted a warm tan. Then I remembered something I had heard long ago, something so dear I had maintained it in my mind. That at the hospice's own care center in West Palm Beach, patients were allowed to bring pets.

"Is that true?" I asked.

"Yes."

"Then that is where I want to go."

Gracie could visit with the children. I imagined the wonderful distraction she would be in those dark hours. Her tail wagging is hypnotic. She is a constant source of delight.

The nurse asked if I wanted a do-not-resuscitate order for my home. An order that specified I was not to be saved. If paramedics rushed to my side in an emergency, all John had to do was show them that DNR.

I had already ordered a medical-alert bracelet that said the same thing, in fourteen-karat gold, of course. Smile.

The hospice nurse stayed past eleven. The children arrived home. I shooed her out the door. We placed the DNR order—a bright yellow paper signed by a doctor—in a drawer, handy but not publicly displayed.

My enrollment in hospice triggered frequent visits by nurses and nurse assistants. Quick visits: vital signs, food intake and outtake. I asked that they remove their hospice IDs when they came to my home so the children would not ask questions. I asked that they try to come during school hours.

I needed help bathing. With weak hands and legs, I could not soap up, could not lather my hair, could not steady myself in the slippery shower.

John had always been my helpmate, but he was still working full-time and already had two boys to bathe.

You know those girls in the locker room who strip down naked and stand there assuredly chatting away?

Yeah, I was not one of those girls.

For most my life, I only donned a bikini in front of a select few. I am modest.

But I felt so sticky and stinky, I agreed to have a stranger bathe me.

I have a claw-foot bathtub, higher off the ground than most, which was a godsend. A hospice nurse assistant helped undress me and lifted me into that tub, filled with warm water and teeming with bubbles.

The assistant was so comfortable, cheerful, and assuring, I began to look forward to her visits. She massaged my scalp—*heaven!*—maneuvered the washcloth just so, dressed me in fresh clothes.

I felt a female communion I had not felt before. One woman bathing another. Slowly, softly. Completely asexual. Talking occasionally. Sharing secrets: the conditioner not placed near the roots of the hair, bony spots where a razor would cut, soft folds that must be scrubbed.

The small things.

Soon the doctor-in-charge learned of my condition: walking with assistance, eating on my own. The doctor asked to see me.

"You're not sick enough for hospice," she told me.

I told the doctor I understood and respected her decision. I had heard that hospice was not just for people at death's door. That's why I signed up. But I wasn't even inside the building yet. I was still outside, walking in the sun.

Three weeks after hospice admitted me, they discharged me.

My sister was thrilled.

"Finally something good happens!" she said.

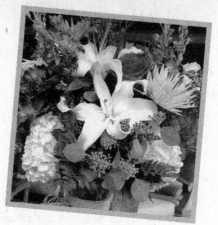

Funeral

Have you ever thought of your funeral? Admit it! Everybody gets one, but only one. What else in life can you say that about?

I thought about my funeral long before I got sick. My, oh my, there must be a dramatic train of black limousines. I'm a sucker for limousines. Fine canapes. Champagne. Tears.

And photos. Not just tacked up on posterboard, but professionally assembled. Set to music. A multimedia presentation.

After every funeral my mother attends, she comments on the number of people in the crowd. "All but the two back pews were filled. Must have been a thousand people there," she would gush. As if that were the barometer of a person's worthiness.

So there must be people at my funeral. Lots of people. My parents have scads of friends, my sister as well. Yes, we probably could raise a crowd.

After I got sick, though, I started caring less. Limousines? Where would they go? Who would even ride in them?

Funerals are for the living, I kept telling myself. And I believe the absolute worst thing that can happen to a human being is to have a child die. So my funeral should be at my parents' church, where hundreds of their friends will surround them with love.

But I am not a Baptist.

I have beliefs. That God exists in each of us.

But religion divides us. That science makes planes, but religion flies them into skyscrapers.

One of my favorite books about belief is *The Tao of Pooh* by Benjamin Hoff. It explains the tenets of Taoism through the simple view of Winnie the Pooh. I quote Hoff's book:

"Rabbit's clever," said Pooh thoughtfully.

"Yes," said Piglet, "Rabbit's clever."

"And he has Brain."

"Yes," said Piglet, "Rabbit has Brain."

There was a long silence.

"I suppose," said Pooh, "that that's why he never understands anything."

Hoff uses Pooh, a calm bear who practices minimal effort, to explain how Taoists achieve peace and power of the mind, in part by not resisting the natural order of the universe.

"That's not a religion!" the Baptists will say.

Which is precisely why I like it.

So here I was, a heathen in the Baptists' eyes. A dying heathen, who sought a funeral in their church.

And not just any funeral, but one that reflected my ecumenical respect for all. I wanted a rabbi, an imam, a Buddhist monk, and a Catholic priest. I wanted each to explain their belief in what happens after death.

I invited First Baptist Church's pastor, Jimmy Scroggins, to my home to request just that: a fully open service. A request almost as outrageous as asking him to host a keg party in his sanctuary.

I told Dad about it. He was appalled, but said nary a word to me, just communicated to Pastor Scroggins that he disagreed with my request. That's one of the first things Pastor Scroggins told me when he arrived at my house: "Your dad doesn't think it's a good idea."

Respectfully, I made my request: "Could a rabbi, imam, monk, and priest be celebrants beside you at my funeral?"

Pastor Scroggins was a charismatic young preacher, a dear holy man devoted to serving the Lord and sharing the word of Jesus Christ. A man of faith. He looked me in the eye and said: "Susan, you can have the Rainbow Coalition stand up and say things about you personally, but not about their beliefs."

He explained that he would not ask to preach at a mosque out of deference to the imam. "It's disrespectful."

He was polite, concerned—and resolute.

I understood. No bitterness. His church, his rules.

I thanked him for coming.

If Dad disagreed anyway, then it should not be. I was trying, trying to inject "me-me-me" all over the funeral, forgetting that funerals are for the living. That the most comforting message my parents could hear on what might well be the worst day of their lives was the one they have heard for decades, the one they believe.

Not the one I do.

Don't overthink things, I tell myself. Be the stuffed bear.

Keep the funeral simple. A few words. A picture-and-music slide show of my life I am preparing with Gwen Berry, a multimedia journalist colleague who offered to help me. A few friends. Just a few. My family. That will be easiest on John. He doesn't like being the center of attention.

He will arrive late, anyway. Smile. My John.

He will have spent the morning wrestling three children into nice clothes. Let them wear shorts, John! Let them enjoy what they can. Whatever is best for the children—my children—that's what I ask of you.

Till then, I will live in the Taoist way: peaceful, not strident about wants or beliefs. I will live in the now.

As Lao Tzu wrote:

> Be content with what you have; rejoice in the way things are.
> When you realize there is nothing lacking, the whole world belongs to you.

I turn away from my iPhone and look at my backyard. Still here. Right now. I text to Aubrey: "Can you come?"

I don't tell him what I want to do: give him a hug. Or more precisely, since I can't hug him very well, I want him to hug me.

Be content. Rejoice. The world belongs to you.

Say those words if you wish, Pastor Scroggins. Or don't. It doesn't matter. Do what you feel is right.

Then donate my body to science.

Science—that I believe in.

Cyprus

June–July

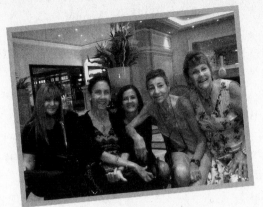

Fearless

We arrived in Cyprus in late June in hundred-degree heat. Hot, yes, but comfortable for my Mediterranean soul.

The first visit, I had been searching. Trying to find a medical explanation, but also a history. Trying to find connections.

This journey was more leisurely. I knew who I was, both my past and my future. This time, I just wanted to spend time with my relatives. Live the culture. Soak in the colors I remembered well: white buildings, green palms and fruit trees, the splays of bougainvillea, fuchsia, red, white, and orange.

This time I brought John, in addition to Nancy. I wanted him to value this land and these people as much as I did, so that the connection would not die with me.

I also brought Ellen, my birth mother. She had asked to come, to explain her actions. Volunteered for what could be quite an inquisition from Panos's relatives.

She had no emotional attachment to Panos. She had

not spoken to him since discovering she was pregnant. But she wanted, I realized, to close her own psychological loop. To address the decision she made in not telling him of me.

I had doubted her once, thinking cowardice kept her—and by extension Panos—from me. Now I saw that she had struggled, and that she was strong.

Fearless!

We went from the airport to the Hilton on the Greek side of Nicosia, a luxury hotel with velvet-upholstered couches, verandas, and a large pool.

There were gifts in our rooms from Panos's family. An antique copy of the book *Peter Pan*—Soulla loves antiques. Jewelry. Chocolates. A book about Cyprus. Phaedra, Soulla's nine-year-old granddaughter, had drawn butterflies on a beautiful card and written "Welcome."

I instantly felt at home.

And pampered. Soulla's son-in-law, Avraam the Operator (who brought Red Bull to Cyprus!), knew the manager of the Hilton. *Voilà*, I had a wheelchair-accessible room on the VIP floor.

"Nice, huh?" John said.

"*Neh*," I replied.

In Greek, *neh* means "yes." So of course I immediately started using it on my poor husband.

"You have to use the bathroom?" he'd ask.

"Neh."

"No?"

"Neh!"

"Stop it!"

Another Greek word I loved was the one for okay: *endaxi*. Or *dox*, for short.

"Dox," I'd reply to John, and he'd roll his eyes.

Then one of my fellow Americans would crack the old "It's all Greek to me" joke. That was when I'd roll my eyes.

My first trip to Cyprus, a mere two years before, I had trundled all over Nicosia. Up the elevator to Soulla's terrace. Up the stairs to centenarian Xenon's apartment. Out to George's house. Around the historic shopping district.

At one point, George had taken us to a beach called Fig Tree Bay. The water was cold, but I didn't want to miss the chance to swim in the Mediterranean. So Nancy (reluctantly, she's a wimp about cold water) and I swam out a couple hundred yards to a floating platform. I pulled myself onto it without help. Lay there for a while, soaking in the colors, sunning, not wanting to leave.

This time, I was marooned at the Hilton. Too weak to walk, too confined in my body to swim on my own.

No bother. The Hilton had a canopied terrace with arches and tables overlooking the pool. A beautiful Mediterranean spot. My spot. Where my relatives could come to me.

And come they did, many nights of the week we were in Cyprus. Glorious gatherings with no expectations or timelines, just jumbles of drinks and food and attempts to seat our party of ten.

This time, it was the children, Phaedra and Anastasia, who charmed me.

I am hyperconscious now that I may scare young children. My wheelchair is all black with large wheels, and I sit, unable to rise or play, slurring and gnarled. I once saw a child turn and bury his face in his mother's legs when he saw me. At that age, I would have been scared too.

But not Phaedra and Anastasia. For them, my chair was a toy. When it was empty, they would hop in and push each other around. John did wheelies with them. Anastasia curled up on his lap one night as we ate dinner.

My old family and new family. Together.

All except Panos. I would have to summon his spirit once again. Would have to journey to him, as he could no longer come to me.

We visited his grave at high noon on an intensely sunny day.

"Odd that we are all wearing black," Ellen said on the way over.

"I meant to," I said. "For the cemetery."

"I didn't think of that. That's not something we do in California," she said.

We stopped to buy flowers. Nancy chose purple flowers called "Immortals," so named because they never wilt, dead or alive.

Panos was buried in his family plot, in a cemetery in the middle of Nicosia—a cemetery so old and crowded that to make room for the newly deceased, they dig up old coffins and bag the bones, then rebury the bag.

An ancient place. A silent place, with cypress trees rising round the living and the dead.

On my first visit, I had stood alone at the graveside. Panos Kelalis. 1932–2002. I could read only his name, written in the Greek alphabet. It felt like our own secret language.

"I am proud to be a part of you," I had telegraphed to him. "I am sad not to have met you."

This time, I came with my husband, relatives, and friend. Nancy placed the Immortals at the grave. I rose from my wheelchair, not wanting the encumbrance. Showing respect and strength. The white marble slab reflected hot light so bright I squinted behind sunglasses.

Our guide Alina—Soulla's daughter, who came from London for our visit—asked the cemetery's Greek Orthodox priest to say a blessing over the grave.

The priest stood facing me in full sun. He had very white hair and a very red, sweating face. He wore a floor-length blue robe with a textile vestment draped around his neck, faded by the sun.

My God, he must be sweltering, I thought.

The priest held an incense burner, a long chain with bells, and an ornate orb on the end containing cinders. He chanted a monotone prayer in Greek. I understood two words and, by his flat affect, that he had said this prayer a thousand times before.

I heard "Panos" and "Theos"—God.

I felt faint in the heat and miasma of death.

I asked to leave, for standing at the grave of my birth father—in cool weather or hot—made me feel no closer to him.

I saw more of him in the ocean painting he loved, in the worry beads he thumbed, in the photos of him, especially as a young adult when he looked like me.

I felt closer to him in the land he considered his home, not the marble tomb where he now lay.

Like all of us, Panos lived in the people he left behind, including me and my children, descendants he never knew.

That night, we convoyed in cars to my friends George and Yioula's beautiful home in the countryside. Their son,

Stelios, had grown a foot since I last saw him, more into the handsome man he was bound to be.

Oh! I hope Marina likes him one day, I thought.

George and Yioula graciously hosted a dinner for the fifteen of us, even though they were leaving on their own vacation the next day.

We sat outside overlooking the surrounding fields. I explained to George I could no longer drink like I used to. My language is so slurred, one drink and I am unintelligible. "But when the talking is over, bring it on!"

Some Cypriot journalists came, friends of George, who is a documentary filmmaker and operator himself. As a former journalist, I felt sorry for them, parachuted into the middle of the saga, struggling to understand.

"Let them ask the questions!" I said, shushing the group, which was overloading them with details.

Nancy had brought gifts and handed them out after dinner. Seven-year-old Anastasia, the smallest child, piped up: "Where is mine?"

I love kids!

I had brought one gift: Panos's Bible. I wanted to present the Bible to Soulla that eve, while I was still strong. I knew I could not speak the words without crying, so I wrote them down on my iPhone and asked Nancy to read. As Nancy took my phone, I began to cry, sniveling so loudly I bowed my head to hide my face. Nancy read:

> Dear Soulla,
>   I will write these words to you, as my voice is weak and my will not to cry much weaker.

At the same time I learned who my birth father, Panos Kelalis, was, I learned he was dead.

Then I parachuted into your life, a true foreigner with an unbelievable story, asking all about him, prying really.

I feared that no one would believe or like me, suspect me of being a gold digger, reject me.

Rather, you responded kindly and shared so much.

Naturally, we talked much of his ex-wife, Barbara, on our last visit. And you mentioned you were disappointed when she came for Panos's funeral and did not bring the family Bible as you asked . . .

"If you meet her, take it!" you said, perhaps in jest, perhaps not.

Barbara remained a curious figure in my mind, not so much for her egregious actions but rather to see who this American princess was who hijacked my father's heart.

I wanted to learn from her something about how he loved.

Nancy read the whole story of Pat's help and Barbara's response. She read:

As I sat on her living room sofa one day, I squinted in the bright sunlight.

"You are squinting just like Panos," she said.

So, in the end, Barbara believed in me. Which

was not nearly as important to me as having the
Bible.

Which I now give to you.

Your goodness has engendered so much more
goodness, peace, and strength in my life. Your
sharing of Panos has helped give me absolute peace
of mind that I do not have a genetic form of ALS,
that I don't have to worry my children will suffer it
one day.

I love the stories of how fearless Panos was. They
help me feel stronger today. . . .

Soulla, you have filled out in my mind who he
was, made me proud to be part of him, made me
sad not to know him. Today, I have stories of his
personality, photos, personal objects of his, thanks
to you and Ellen.

I have an image of him I admire much. I hope,
hope to meet him on the other side of life.

I am not fearful of death. I am fearless.

Thank you. Efcharisto.

Soulla sat in stunned silence.

Nadia, the spitfire, asked to see the Bible. "No, I don't
think that's the one," she chirped right away.

Avraam inspected it and discovered something Pat,
Nancy, and I had missed. A highlighted passage, in fluorescent yellow, about how a wife is to do the husband's bid-
ding.

Ack! It's Barbara's Bible!

"Well, it's the thought that counts!" I said to the group.

We all had a good laugh. And in that moment, the embarrassment turned into another memory, another story to share under the Chickee hut like wine.

Stelios, George's son, invited us to a piano recital inside. He played "The Star-Spangled Banner." Anastasia stood by, conducting. I about had Marina married off to Stelios by the end of it. Roll your eyes, Marina, but 'tis true.

George, Nancy, and I had been students together in the University of Florida's graduate journalism program. Nancy and I had posed as actors in some short films George had to make in his TV production course.

George had found the films and played them for us. There was Nancy twenty years younger, the only difference her hair three times bushier then.

And there was me. So very, very different. My hair blond and bushy, my face plump, not sunken as it is now. And my hands.

The video was of me making a Greek salad. The camera zoomed in on my hands, holding the tomato, cucumber, and onion.

My fingers nimble and thin, the natural nails long and smooth.

Fingers now curling as the muscles weaken. Nails untamed and often dirty, as I am unable to manicure them myself.

What do I do?

What do I do in such bright-line moments, where my handicap whomps me over the head?

Dwell in what there remains to be grateful for.

My hands are snarled, but I can still touch. I cannot hold,

but I can feel. I have my connection to the world, which ALS will never take away.

I had one more journey to take in Cyprus. A journey home. A trip full of sights. Sounds. Tastes. Touch. A journey to delight my senses.

Senses forever mine.

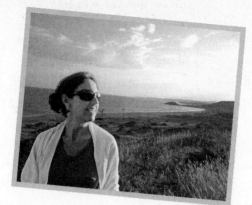

Turtle Beach

On my first visit to Cyprus, Soulla had told me of an extraordinary day she and Panos spent together around 1996. They had visited sites from their childhood in northern Cyprus: first a beach Panos had loved, then a monastery.

Soulla showed me a photo of Panos standing in a breezeway at the monastery, framed by arches.

"I want to go there," I said.

For that is how you summon spirit. To go.

I did not realize the impact of what I had asked.

Since 1974, Cyprus has been a divided island, with a Greek side and a Turkish one. Even the capital Nicosia is divided. As rigidly split as East and West Berlin once were, so is Nicosia today.

The war between Greece and Turkey, two nations with a long history on the island, had been intense. Both nations sent their armies. Many died. Tens of thousands more were uprooted from their homes.

Every Cypriot remembers those days, even the children who have only heard the tales.

"My mother was hanging clothes on the line," a Turkish friend, Firat, told us, recounting a Greek bombing run. "She ran out of her flip-flops, she was so scared."

Avraam was thirteen years old when the Turkish army neared his home. He, his three siblings, and his parents got in the family car and headed for safety in the pine forest of a mountain range hours away.

"My father said, 'We will stay here tonight,' " Avraam recounted. "And I said, 'Where here?' "

They slept in the pine forest for a month, expecting to return home any day.

They never could.

The United Nations brokered a demarcation line, the Green Line. Greeks to the south in the Republic of Cyprus; Turks to the north in the self-declared (and never internationally recognized) Turkish Republic of Northern Cyprus. No one could cross between the two.

The island was divided—as divided as I was from my birth father, the man I sought to know.

Panos and Soulla were Greek Cypriots from the north. In 1996, neither had been to their childhood homes in more than twenty years. Then Panos received a rare opportunity.

A renowned pediatric surgeon, he saved the life of a Turkish minister's son. The minister, grateful, asked what he could do for Panos in return.

Panos asked that he and Soulla be allowed to cross the border and visit sites from their childhood.

They were granted one day, under military escort. That's how strict was the divide.

By the time of my first visit in 2010, tensions had eased. The Green Line remained, but George and Yioula had been allowed take me across the border for a day.

I had not understood how difficult this was for them. Asking Greek Cypriots to cross to the Turkish side was akin to asking a Cuban exile to take you back to Cuba. The sense of loss, both personal and cultural, was profound.

As we crossed the border, Yioula summarized her feelings in a whisper: "A thousand sighs."

On that first trip, we drove past Yioula's childhood house in Famagusta, a place usurped by a Turkish family. George had tried to dissuade her, but Yioula had been adamant. She looked intently, but spoke not a word.

Afterward, we headed across a desolate landscape to the eastern shore of the island, following the path Panos had taken with Soulla in 1996. Like them, we had only hours. I had not known the story when I arrived, and I could only fit a day into my schedule.

On this second trip, I was determined to return to northern Cyprus. To immerse myself, unlike the first time, in the places Panos had loved. In the Saint Andreas monastery, from which the medal I now wore as a necklace—Panos's medal—had come.

And on Turtle Beach, where, as Soulla told it, Panos had taken off his shoes and danced on the golden sand, his arms over his head, twirling with joy.

The eastern Karpaz Peninsula, where Panos was raised, is hilly, rocky, dusty, and desolate. Few people live in the region, especially since the Turkish invasion, and the land is not cultivated as on the Greek side. You can drive and drive the lone road and see nothing but rock and brush, brown fields and bramble.

Then you emerge a hundred feet above a cove, where sapphire blue water melds to teal.

A dozen turns, then back again through miles of brown fields and bramble before another bend reveals a larger cove, where sapphire melds to teal and teal to turquoise.

A hand-lettered sign in the middle of nowhere indicated we had arrived: "Hasan's Turtle Beach Ok for cars."

We turned onto a sand road that wended down a hill toward the shore. About halfway down, we pulled up to an open-air eatery, the only building, and parked.

Then stepped out into a postcard.

The day was so clear, we could see the mountains of Turkey forty miles away. There was not one cloud. Sun shone on every inch of the panorama, lighting the expanse of Mediterranean before us a brilliant blue.

At the oceanside, I have so often marveled at the colors.

The Pacific's deep violet, seen from the edge of a cliff in Hawaii with John.

Every shade of aquamarine in the waters around the Bahamas, the shallow flats like blue beach glass as Nancy and I flew overhead.

The Atlantic Ocean, my ocean, has more hues of green than blue. In my mind, green is good for bedrooms, but not oceans. An opinion stemming from childhood memories of endless days afloat in blue, blue pools. If a pool was greenish, it was dirty.

But the color of the Mediterranean at Turtle Beach.

Oh, the color!

Not a navy blue nor a royal blue. A sapphire blue. A jewel with hints of teal and turquoise, the full spectrum spreading for miles beyond a gold-tinted beach.

I asked to be parked in my wheelchair right there by the car, under a tree, wanting just to sit and sear that image into my mind.

I could see why Panos adored the spot. I adored it too.

The water was more than a football field of sand away. I told John I wanted to remain there and not go down to the beach.

Hasan (the manager of the eatery) and John lifted my wheelchair over bumps on the path to the thatch-roofed restaurant. We ordered beers and kebabs, out of the sun but squarely in the scenery.

The beach could have held thousands of people. There were perhaps twenty there.

The others left me and went down to the shore to swim. From my vantage point, they looked like specks in the sand.

I thought of that quote by Isaac Newton, when he compared himself to a boy playing at the seashore, focused on the shells, "whilst the great ocean of truth lay all undiscovered before me."

I thought how fine my view at the top was, where I could see the color, the expanse of the sea. I actively tried to make it okay not to be able to get down there and swim and dance on the sand.

That is the secret I learn more of every day. Not to want things I cannot have or cannot do.

Remove the want, and you remove the pain.

John and Nancy returned from their swim. "How was the water?" I asked.

"Perfect!" John said. Calm, clear, and warm.

John said the view underwater was boring, nothing but sand. No fish. No mollusks. Not even rocks.

Nancy gushed about the underwater light, like a kaleidoscope of blue and yellow glass.

Perspective. It's all perspective.

We had more beer and kebabs and finally, reluctantly, left in the late afternoon to drive to our hotel on the Turkish side of the border. We did so mostly in silence, save for periodic eruptions of laughter.

Nancy, operating the right-side-drive van (Cyprus had long been a British territory, and they still drove on the British side of the road), instinctively expected the turn signal to be on the left side of the wheel. Each time she flipped it, she turned on the windshield wipers.

They'd swish across the dusty glass. "Okay, I am going to concentrate!" Nancy said. "And not do that again."

She did it the whole drive.

A slight haze set in. The sea turned more black than blue. The sun set over the ocean, reflecting so intensely there appeared a bump in the horizon where the light met the water, as if the sun was pulling a wave into its light.

The evening haze colored the mountains a gray blue. At one point we saw six fingerling slopes, each subsequent one a paler blue-gray, a shadow of the others.

An extraordinary sight to end our extraordinary day, tracing the footsteps of an extraordinary man.

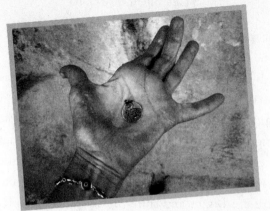

Saint Andreas

The monastery sat on a cape extending into the Mediterranean Sea. Apostolos Andreas. A place of history. A pilgrimage for the Greek Orthodox faithful, who sought the healing power of Saint Andreas.

Author Colin Thubron, in his book *Journey into Cyprus*, noted that as early as 1191 AD, an abbey had stood on the site. Today a fifteenth-century chapel covers its healing wells. Legend has it that the water sprang beneath the feet of Saint Andreas as he landed on the shore.

In 1972, when Thubron wrote, the giant square of huts around the monastery accommodated visitors by the hundreds. "For St. Andreas is a great miracle-worker, and this is the Lourdes of Cyprus."

Thubron described a carnival atmosphere as people flocked there for blessings and miracles. He witnessed a throng of baptisms being held with the "drive of an industry," the faithful lifting their children to kiss the icons there.

That must have been the Saint Andreas of Panos's childhood, the memory he loved and sought.

But by 1996, Saint Andreas was not the monastery of Panos's youth. When the Turks invaded in 1974, dividing the country and cutting eastern Cyprus off from its Greek population, churches became a casualty. Visit a village in the Karpaz region today and you will see plants growing out of church roofs and cat and pigeon dung coating its sanctuary.

There are bright and shiny mosques now, built for the new population, their minarets visible above village homes.

The Saint Andreas monastery was not spared. Walls were crumbling, revealing ancient stones pitted by neglect. The huts that had housed pilgrims were filled with debris. On the day of our visit, feral cats, skinny dogs, and two wild donkeys were the only other pilgrims.

"That's the most depressed-looking cat I've ever seen," Soulla's daughter Alina said.

The archway where Panos had stood for his photograph looked forsaken. Plaster chipping away. Paint flaking. A desolate place, not the happy place it had seemed with my birth father standing within it.

Yet I smiled, as I could feel him here, in this place he loved.

I could imagine the monastery full of the faithful, Panos among them, kissing the golden icons, standing close as the priest chanted and swung the bell-adorned orb full of burning incense.

I imagined smelling the sweet incense on Panos as he kissed me good night.

That is how you summon spirit.

That is how you close a divide.

The holy waters of San Andreas still flowed, despite the monastery's decrepit state. Down many steps, near the sea-shore, was a font.

I asked John to help me to where the holy water flows. He carried me in his arms down a set of stairs, breathing heavily, trying not to slip on the worn stone steps.

I had visited the Saint Andreas Monastery in 2010, on my first visit to Cyprus. We arrived in the late afternoon. I had time for little more than a photograph, in the exact spot where Panos had stood for his photo, and a walk to the font.

As the sun fell away in the west, I placed Panos's Saint Andreas medallion, the one in his pocket when he died, in my withered left hand. I held it under the stream of cool water.

"Hello, God," I prayed. "Please solve this mystery. Please let it be something other than ALS. Please let my children keep their mother. For they have done nothing wrong."

I took a photograph of my hand with the medallion in the palm, water running over it.

Then stood there, silently. Hoping.

On this second visit, I thought I might pray for a miracle.

Yes, I believe in miracles, I concluded on the drive to the monastery.

I had only to look at my mother. She was a miracle, to have been so close to death and to be alive today.

Yes, I believe in miracles.

But I didn't expect a miracle.

Nor did I feel I deserved one.

My mother had been a faithful worshipper all her life. I had not. My mother had always been mindful of God, while I had not.

John set me down to rest himself about twenty stairs away from the holy water font. "That's okay," I told him, "You don't need to take me further."

A full moon rose behind me above the Mediterranean. I could barely turn to see it.

The trip to Cyprus accelerated my weakening. I could no longer turn my body. I could no longer hold things in my right hand. My left foot for the first time entirely buckled when I put weight on it without my brace. My speech was so slurred I was reluctant to talk.

"So sad," I slurred, as I sat with John, looking over the decrepit monastery.

He looked at his watch. "It's 7:40," he replied, misunderstanding my remark.

The moon rose higher over the Mediterranean, and the monastery fell toward darkness. Alina drove our car across the gravel parking lot to pick me up. *Crunch, crunch, crunch,* as I slowly stepped to the car, John holding me upright. I was grateful I could walk at all.

We arrived back late at the Theresa Hotel, tired and hungry.

We had found the hotel in 2010, as we drove along the coast near Yalusa, the Greek village where Panos was raised. No one had been at the desk when we rang the bell, but an older man soon came, carrying snails. He had been out hunting for them.

He was Erdogan, the owner of the inn. He had known Panos's father, a teacher at the elementary school.

"Your friend grandfather came from Karava near Kyrenia," Erdogan later e-mailed Nancy. "He loved Yalusa. He rent a house and continue his life, a teacher at elementary school. He had good contact with villager. He help them to make tobacco. They build big factory to save the tobacco. After he worked in organization for to give money to the villager. The Yalusa people loved him."

The Theresa Hotel was a no-star inn, with white plastic furniture and bare lightbulbs and mismatched sheets. But its open-air restaurant sat in a five-star spot, on a hill overlooking the sea.

This corner of Earth was luminous.

We ordered a seafood mezze, expecting subpar fare in the spare surroundings. Sorry, Erdogan, but 'tis true.

A tattooed waiter in a muscle shirt brought the plates. First, a fresh chopped salad of ruby red tomato and cucumber. Then a lentil and rice salad. A bulghur wheat salad. Fresh hummus, yogurt, and pita. Black salty olives. Beer.

Then the main course began. First, a mound of prawns, each one as big as a fist, their antennae curling over the edge of the plate. Fresh fried calamari. A pile of small silver fish. There was no room left on the table.

We ate and ate, passing the plates. John peeled the prawns for me. We mastered an eating system in Cyprus, where he fed me at every meal. Rather than preparing a small bite and waiting for me to swallow, he left me chewing and returned to his meal. I softly tapped him when I was ready for another.

Tap, tap, tap. I tapped away, delighted with the meal.

We were stuffed when out came the waiter with a pile of filleted fish and lobsters.

Tap, tap, tap!

The meal ended with a platter of watermelon and plums. We sat, drinking, smoking, talking.

We had hired a two-person Cypriot film crew to film our trip to the north. Stella, the sound tech, said she would like to share something with us, a song.

Now, Stella is a wisp of a young woman with long, thin limbs, high-top sneakers, and a boyish haircut. One place we went, she was mistaken for a child.

On Erdogan's terrace, she closed her eyes and opened her mouth and sang a cappella. Sang in a voice I could not believe came from that fragile body. Sang in perfect pitch a song in Greek about a woman whose sailor love was leaving for sea.

I understood not a word. Yet could have listened forever.

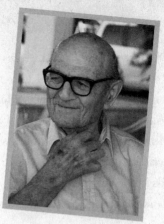

The Old Man of Karpaz

Earlier in the day, in the same white plastic chair where Stella sang, had sat another extraordinary soul, a man named Savas.

When we booked the reservation, Erdogan had volunteered to help find people in neighboring villages who knew Panos or his father, Petros, the village teacher.

"The elder of the Greek village, the Old Man of the Karpaz, he knew them," Erdogan said. "I will bring him to you."

Before we went to the monastery, the eighty-two-year-old Savas appeared. He wore thick black eyeglasses and walked with a cane. He had one upper tooth.

"I am getting my teeth Monday," he said, beaming.

Savas chose to remain in his Greek village after the Turkish invasion. He became the area's consummate diplomat, Erdogan said, engaging the Turks, promoting peace, hosting the United Nations relief workers who supplied the village.

Savas spoke Greek, Turkish, and British English very well.

So well, in fact, he corrected Nancy's pronunciation of the word *daughter*.

"Ah, that's right, you're American." He smiled.

Savas had gone to school with Panos. I asked if Panos had been a cut-up in class. I had been one: switching the clock, trimming ponytails, and Nancy's favorite, dangling pencils from my nostrils during math lessons.

"No, no. Panos was a good boy. A teacher's son," Savas said.

Savas knew my grandfather, Petros, and grandmother, Julia. Now remember, Julia was the mustachioed woman I once mistook in a photo for a man.

"Does Susan look like Panos?" Nancy asked Savas.

"She looks like her grandmother," he said.

Nancy and I burst out laughing. She moved in for the kill.

"Was she a pretty woman?"

"She was . . . a lady," Savas said swiftly.

Nancy and I laughed uncontrollably. Alina, who recollects as a child being scared of the mustachioed Julia, silently smiled.

I switched subjects, interested in Savas's life as a refugee in his own home.

Erdogan had said there was something Savas wouldn't tell us. That he lost a son in the war. Truly lost him. That his son never came home, dead or alive.

Savas told us that his Greek village was now sixty-eight people, down from hundreds. The youngest villager was forty-two years old, finally married but unable to have children.

I asked Savas if he was happy he'd remained.

"A million percent happy," he said.

He expressed no bitterness, no hate, no blame, though he had watched his village dwindle away and lost his son.

I will never forget that attitude.

Thank you, Old Man of the Karpaz. Thank you.

I leave Cyprus, the physical island and place in my heart, with your outlook in mind.

New York City

City

July

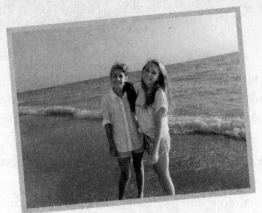

Kardashians

My daughter Marina was crackin' me up describing her Cuban-American friend's mother, Alex, and Alex's various beliefs.

For example, Alex believes that if you talk on a cell phone when the battery is low, you will get cancer. And if you go to bed with your hair wet, you will get pneumonia. And if you swim in a pool with leaves in it, you will get some god-awful disease.

Marina has been a vegetarian for years now—her choice, not mine—and this horrifies Alex, who is convinced it will impair Marina's fertility.

"She told me I am going to have to put yogurt in my vagina one day," Marina said.

Marina and her friend, Lizzy, aren't permitted to sleep together in Lizzy's queen-size bed out of fear they might become "lesbos," as Marina says, making quotation marks with her fingers.

One morning Lizzy's father found them sleeping in the

bed. "He asked us if we had kissed," Marina said, screwing her face up in a WTF expression.

Marina's eyes widen and a true look of horror comes across her face, though, when she says the following: "They make Lizzy clean the whole house!"

Here at the Wendels', a primary source of arguments is Miss Marina's utter lack of tidiness.

Her bedroom and bathroom often look as if drag-queen burglars have rifled through every drawer, tried on every piece of clothing, opened every makeup container, brushed their teeth, then left their spittle in the sink and the flat-iron singeing the vanity.

When I could walk and yell—I can no longer project my voice enough to make loud noises—I did a lot of stormin' into her room, scoopin' up scattered items and hollerin', "I'll give these to a kid who will take care of them!"

I distinctly remember standing in front of my children yelling, "Stop yelling!!"

No more.

Now I am more namby-pamby, another silver lining of this LouG mess. I sit stuck in my Chickee hut, unable to see the jumble in Marina's room, getting my Zen on and mulling how you can't fight nature. You can't fight the messy habits of a teenage girl.

And I can't fight what is happening to me. There is no cure for ALS.

(Which, by the way, is absurd. Seventy-three years after Lou Gehrig's famous speech, there's still nothing. Absurd! I mean, my phone can talk to me. We can play remote control cars on Mars. But we can't figure out how to keep nerves alive.)

"What will be, will be," I tell myself.

And in comes John, hollering: "I can't believe you let her go to the beach with her room looking like that!"

"Don't fight nature," I calmly reply.

"Susan! It's unsanitary!"

I have lapsed so in that department of parenting. The badger-the-heck-outta-your-kids-to-make-them-better-neater-sanitary-people department. I can travel to Hungary and Cyprus, but I cannot walk into my daughter's room to tell her to pick up her dirty shirt.

I have saddled my poor husband with the job.

John, formerly one of the most even-tempered Joes you will ever meet, now has near-daily meltdowns trying to get the kids to pick up wrappers, put their clothes and dishes away, or help unload the dishwasher.

A fiber bar wrapper left on the sofa can result in a fifteen-minute brouhaha, beginning: "I told you not to eat on the sofa!"

This morning, John awoke Aubrey by banging on a pot and ordering him out of bed to pick up said wrapper.

Poor John. I have let things slide and slide, unwilling to ask the children to do the things I used to do. Now making him be the disciplinarian. The parent who walks in the room—now that I can't walk—and tells them no.

"Don't you dare make Marina feel like she has to be the mom," I tell John all the time.

Mercifully, Marina is fourteen years old. Which is to say, she is living on another planet. She is often too busy with her friends to think about me.

Much of the time, she may as well be riding in that remote control car on Mars.

I was reminded of this the other eve when she bopped in the room and asked if she could change the TV channel to the reality show *Keeping Up with the Kardashians*. "Sure," I said, eager to share something with her.

I prefer *Law & Order* or *Frozen Planet* or perhaps *My Big Fat Gypsy Wedding*, the last to marvel at how the young women in that community dress like prostitutes. The gypsy wedding show at least has a cheap gaudy quotient going for it. But the Kardashians?

Marina watched rapt with attention as a bunch of gorgeous women whose names all begin with "K" and their emasculated spouses fought, and the K's played jokes like hiding one another's Ferraris, and K-Mom flitted in and out of their mansion, too busy with her booming business to cook dinner for her children, while driving with the K-kids in her sports car, flipping birds and cursing at other drivers.

Marina was fascinated.

"Whyever would you want to watch this show?" I asked.

"What's not to love?" she answered.

"What do you love about it? What? Help me understand."

"Oh, Mom, you are so cute."

Yes, Marina often says I am cute, as she bops from one room to another, dyeing her hair or raiding my closet, passing me in my chair as I try to feed myself from a tray like a two-year-old.

"You are soooo cute," she says.

And my soul smiles.

I am glad I am cute to her.

"I want to take you on a trip," I tell her. One that she will remember long after I'm gone. I want a way into her world, at least for a few days. I don't tell her that part.

"Where would you like to go?"

Her eyes pop open wide. She smiles. "Calabasas, California. To meet the Kardashians."

She is not kidding.

Years ago, I saw the movie *Life Is Beautiful*, about a man in a concentration camp with his young son. The man reinvents the experience for the child, hiding the horror in humor and fantasy. Hiding the horror with his spirit.

That is what I try to do every day with ALS. For a long time, we did not say the name around the kids, because then they are one Google away from the horror.

Early on, a psychologist advised John and me not to talk about my disease with the children. Children ask, he told us, when they are ready.

Marina has hardly asked a thing.

I hope hope hope I am doing the right thing. That I am doing what I should for my children. I wonder if one day it all will backfire, if Marina will be disappointed that we did not discuss my disease or what dying young taught me.

I hope not.

She is only fourteen. And perfectly herself.

I am an awful prognosticator of human behavior. I never ever woulda guessed that humans would pay $5 for a cup of coffee if you gave it an Italian name. Or pay big bucks to stand in the sun and watch race cars drive around in circles. Or watch *Keeping Up with the Kardashians*.

But this I do know, or at least I think I do: the stronger I am, the stronger my children will be.

Wesley thinks it's the coolest thing that I now eat on a tray just like he does at school. He's sheltered, too, by Asperger's.

"Mom, can I use your tray?" he asks.

"Of course," I answer.

He plops beside me. "This is cool," he says.

He watches intently as I take an olive and lift it slowly toward my mouth.

"Do you like Lilo or Stitch?" he asks.

I look at him, chewing slowly. He smiles. Yes, my son, this is very cool indeed.

And Marina?

I would have taken you to Calabasas, California, in a second, my love. But you can't just walk up to the Kardashians—even if you still can walk.

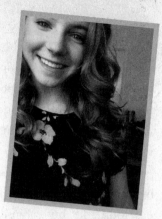

Marina's Trip

The trip to New York came together in a second, right in the beauty parlor, while my hairstylist was coloring my hair.

Kerri is more than a hairstylist, she is a friend. We have known each other for ten years. Our daughters have been good friends since kindergarten. Our sons used to carpool to school.

She had been divorced from her husband for as long as I had known her. Now she was getting married to her girlfriend Pam.

Pam is a microbiologist. An amiable, sweet-souled scientist adept at interacting with people as well as petri dishes. Kerri was over-the-moon happy to have found her. She didn't have to tell me that—though she did, a hundred times.

I could see it in the bouncy way she slathered on my dye.

Kerri is what I call a hug-the-housekeeper girl—so affectionate she hugs everyone, including my housekeeper Yvette, each time she comes over. When she's happy, you know.

During the wait for the hair dye to glom onto my gray, Kerri told me details of her upcoming wedding.

It would be in New York, where same-sex marriage is legal. Her dress would be ice-blue, Pam's dress black. Reception at Pam's sister's house in Hackensack, New Jersey. Cupcakes made by the Cake Boss, with hydrangea flowers because hydrangeas look like butterflies. Kerri's deceased mother loved butterflies.

There were a host of other details planned to memorialize their loved ones lost. Their bouquets would be mementos of those souls. The coins Grandpa always rubbed together; the flowers Grandma made with fabric from her old dresses; a small photo of the baby that died; a piece of beach glass—ice blue and tear-shaped—that they found one day when Kerri was badly missing her dead brother.

In her shoes, I would have been hyperfocused on the perfect bouquet: purple roses atop short stems bound in just-the-right-color ribbon. And here were Kerri and Pam, their chief concern to hold the dead in their hands.

I was so moved, I invited myself to the wedding.

Then I remembered that the year before, Marina had wanted desperately go on a school trip to New York. Until I told her she'd have to improve her school grades, that is. Then she decided it was too much trouble.

"Do you want to go to New York City?" I asked Marina that night. "Kerri is getting married there."

"Sure," Marina said.

"Is there anywhere else you'd rather go?"

Marina smiled. I gotta brag, she has the prettiest smile. Calabasas, anyone? "No, Mom," she said. "New York is good."

"We can shop."

"Really!" Now she was excited.

"We can go to a Broadway show. One with trumpets. And maybe . . . Kleinfeld's?"

Marina and I loved the television show *Say Yes to the Dress*: the bridezillas playing dress-up at the famous bridal shop Kleinfeld's, the fashion, the drama, the families coming together. I told her so many times: "Baby, we're going to Kleinfeld's for your wedding dress one day."

And I always keep my promises.

At least the ones that mean something.

"Okay," Marina said.

"Maybe you can try on a dress."

"Mommmm! I'm only fourteen."

The previous weekend, Marina had gone to an eighth-grade dance. Her first. For hours upon hours, she shopped for the dress, the earrings, the shoes, the right shade of foundation, and then a second trip for the right shade of lipstick. That's my girl!

She looked gorgeous, mature yet young. With her first pair of high heels on, she walked like a newborn pony, her legs too long for her body, unsteady. She was the vision of youth, that self-conscious smile.

She hadn't even started high school yet, and I was suggesting a wedding dress.

"Just for fun, Marina. Haven't you ever wanted to see that store?"

"I guess so." She perked up. "And then we can shop."

"Of course."

I didn't tell her what I was thinking at that moment. That she was right on the cusp. That she could be anybody she wanted to be.

That I would not see the woman she became. I would not see her graduate, or listen to her senior concert. I would probably never meet her date to prom.

I didn't tell her how much I wanted this. To visit Kleinfeld's. To watch my daughter walk out of the dressing room in white silk and see her, suddenly, ten years in the future, in the back room before her wedding, in a moment I will never share.

No expectations, I told myself.

Don't make Marina's life about you.

In New York, I promised myself, we would do what came naturally. Marina would try on as many dresses as she wished, but only as many as she wished, even if that was none. I would not ask anything of her. I would not have expectations. I would not force my daughter to do anything she didn't want to do.

I realized long ago, when I was diagnosed, that I can't force anything. Get your Zen on, Susan. What will be will be.

We would not buy a dress. Some journalist wrote that later: that Marina and I were going to New York to buy a wedding dress.

That writer: what a man! No woman in her right mind would buy a wedding dress at least a decade before her marriage. No mother would force that on her daughter. Fashions morph. Times change.

I simply wanted to make a memory.

I wanted to see my beautiful daughter on her wedding day. I wanted to glimpse the woman she will be.

Maybe I would cry. Mothers cry, right? But I knew I would laugh, too. Because I would be with my Marina. I would be imagining her happy.

That's the memory I wanted to make.

When my only daughter thinks of me on her wedding day, as I hope she will, I want her to think of my smile when I say to her at Kleinfeld's, "You are beautiful, my child."

"You are so cute, Mom," Marina said, bringing me back to the moment. "We can totally go to Kleinfeld's."

She took a strand of hair that had come out of my ponytail and tucked it behind my ear. Something I could no longer do, even when the hair tickled my nose.

She put her arm around me in a teenage almost-hug. I patted it with my curled fingers.

One moment, perfect like that.

She jumped up, that Marina smile on her face. "Can I have some money? Casey is going to get ice cream."

"Sure, honey," I said. "Get my wallet out of my purse."

She did.

"New York," I said, smiling as she slipped $20 into her back pocket. "Bring me the change, please."

"Oh, Mom," Marina said. "You are so cute."

And she was gone.

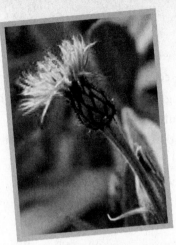

Tattoos

I don't know how the subject of tattoos came up. Never had one. Never wanted one.

But we were in the Chickee hut. Stephanie. John. A few friends. Marina.

Things get said under the Chickee. Lots of things. It seems to have a diuretic effect: words just run out of people's mouths.

So I suppose it was a joke. We were going to Kleinfeld's, a TLC show. Why not NYInk? A Brooklyn tattoo shop with its own show on TLC as well?

Sheesh. For people who lived mostly without cable, we sure were influenced by television.

"I'll get one here," I said, laughing.

"Where, Mom? On your upper leg?"

Arrgh. I could no longer bend down to point.

"No, my ankle. It will say—" I stopped to get control of my tongue. I have to do that for big words. " 'Serendipity.' "

"What's that?" Marina asked.

Serendipity. Good luck. An aptitude for making desirable discoveries by accident.

The word I would use to describe my whole life.

"Look it up," I said.

"Oh, Mom," Marina said, rolling her eyes. "I don't look things up. You know that."

Only your friend Casey doing his crazy butt-dance on YouTube, I thought. In a blond wig, no less.

I didn't think much of the conversation until a few days later, when Marina came up to my chair and sat down on the arm, like she often does. She took a strand of my hair and tucked it softly behind my ear. I love that.

"I really want to get a tattoo in New York," Marina said.

Oh, brother. What have I done?

"A blue cornflower on my ankle."

She smiled, but I could tell she was serious.

"Why, sweetie?"

"Because that's the symbol of ALS."

I guess she does look things up. And knows.

Of course she does. She's a smart girl. I cannot shelter her. She knows my diagnosis. My future. That there is no cure. That the end is near.

And she wants to keep me close. She wants me with her, forever under her skin.

She almost got me. She really did.

Until John, the voice of reason, said: "No tattoos, Susan. My gosh. She's fourteen."

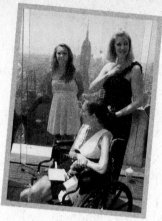

Support

The Marriott Marquis is a huge hotel, right on Times Square. If there's a place on earth that is the antithesis of Turtle Beach, I realized, with its sapphire waters and empty sand, it is Times Square.

There are people everywhere, even in the road. No cars allowed here.

The buildings tower overhead. Every store seems to have lights thirty feet high. The tower where they drop the New Year's Eve ball is covered with a stack of electronic billboards. The police station sits right in the middle of the road.

Did I mention the people dressed in full-body cartoon character suits, begging coins in exchange for photos with kids?

The main entrance to the Marriott Marquis is through a short tunnel and across four rows of taxis. Inside, people wander in all manner of outfits, from saris to cowboy hats. There is a bank of elevators to the eighth-floor lobby, then a central atrium forty floors high.

In the middle, the round glass elevators whisk people upward, again and again. The elevators look like pneumatic tubes. The kind Mom used to put checks in when she drove to the service window at the bank. Then I'd get a lollipop back.

The kind of tubes in movies with old mailrooms.

I loved it.

I had not been to New York City since 1988, when I was an intern at the United Nations for a summer. I lived in a room without a bathroom at the Martha Washington, a women-only boarding house with rats as large as cats.

I loved that summer. I worked hard at the UN. Walked the city. Became friends with interns from all over the world. I rode the subway with them to Queens and mysterious, far-out Brooklyn neighborhoods to eat their native cuisines.

Now I was getting a different view of New York. Not just from two feet lower, because of my wheelchair, but from the view of a mother with a daughter gawking at every store.

Not to mention Stephanie stumbling along beside us, still recovering after white-knuckling the entire three-hour flight from Florida.

We'd added an extra day to the trip, at the request of my publisher. At first I was leery. I wanted this time to be about Marina. But a New York publisher was putting us up for the night and paying to change our plane tickets. As Marina would say: "What's not to love!"

So first stop was across town for an interview at the publisher.

While I worked, Marina was taken on a quick tour by her "two gay dads," my agent Peter and his friend. (An inside joke—they are both straight and married.) They went to the Plaza Hotel—"Wesley used to be OB-sessed with Eloise," Marina told them—Central Park, and a Japanese department store called Uniqlo, which Marina found too weird for shopping.

Then I had an interview with an editor from *People* magazine. Nicest woman ever.

After, we tried to visit Serendipity, a famous ice cream shop. There are steep steps and no wheelchair access. I sat outside, enjoying the sun, writing, while Marina and Stephanie went inside. Someone came by and offered me a dollar.

Marina and Stephanie brought me iced hot chocolate, the Serendipity special. I drank it outside in the sun. Perfect.

Back at the hotel, I gave Marina my credit card. She went shopping on Times Square. Yes, I let Marina shop alone in New York City. You can't helicopter-parent. You have to trust your children and the world.

Just the week before, Marina and her friend had been jumping off a bridge into our local lake. It was only ten feet high, but some parents wouldn't let their children go.

Who was I to say no? Hadn't I jumped off bridges all my life? Yes, literally, when I was a teen. In fact, I jumped off the exact same bridge.

But also when I went to Hungary. When I went to Colombia. When I married John on a whim. When I opened the letter from my birth mama.

But what about the alligators? There are always alligators in Florida waterways, right? No, only the possibility of alligators, and you can't quail at possibilities.

John himself had gone in that same lake the year before, when Marina's retainer had somehow flown out of her mouth and into the water while we were standing in Steph's back-yard. He and Marina dug around in the weedy water for half an hour, and if cautious John thinks the water is safe enough for the two of them to prowl, then how can I deny my daughter a little fun?

(They found the retainer, by the way, buried in the weeds.)

"Be careful with this card." That's all I told Marina before she skipped out the door. I wasn't worried she'd get lost or spend too much or endanger herself.

I wasn't worried about pickpockets, either. My only worry was that her jeans were so snug, the pressure on her pocket would catapult the card right into the air.

How oh how did skintight become such a fashion?

She was back for the party that evening. It was a reception thrown by Peter in the rotating restaurant on the forty-somethingth floor of the Marriott Marquis. Folks from the publisher and from Peter's agency. Charles Passy, the friend who blogged about me in the *Wall Street Journal*. David Smith, the lawyer who had shown Peter the article. Two movie people who wanted to make a film about my life.

"They came all the way from Los Angeles to meet you," Peter told me later, clearly impressed.

I went to bed right after the party. When it takes you fifteen minutes, and all your strength, just to sit on the toilet, you tend to get tired.

The last thing I remember was Marina standing at the window of our hotel room, looking at the Times Square lights.

When I woke the next morning, everything seemed the same. The city truly had not slept. It just went on and on.

We went with it. To breakfast. To more shopping for Marina.

Pam and Kerri's wedding was at noon at Rockefeller Center, so we decided to walk the eight blocks. Stephanie pushed me in my wheelchair.

We arrived early enough to roll around the Rock. We gazed at the strangely muted brown skyscrapers. At the famous ice rink, now filled with tables for the summer. There were a hundred flags, at least, from around the world.

And fifteen stairs, with no ramp. Stephanie helped me up, one step at a time, while Marina carried my wheelchair. By the time I reached the top, we were sweating in our wedding attire. Even me in my sleeveless black-and-white dress, the one Stephanie had helped me pick out a few weeks before.

"Let's go," I said. "It's time."

The wedding was at Top of the Rock, the observation deck. There was an actual red carpet on the sidewalk outside the door. The wedding guests clustered inside.

The brides arrived. They kissed everyone. Handed out gifts. An efficient woman herded us into a special corridor, then around the tourist line to the elevator.

The elevator was bedlam. Twenty-something people sucked upward so fast our ears popped. A video on the ceiling flashed rapidly moving images, with loud music.

We arrived with a whoosh of hydraulic brakes. The music and images stopped. The other wedding guests started to file off.

"Look," Steph whispered, pointing up.

There, on the ceiling of the elevator, was a ladybug. It had been hidden by the throbbing video.

I thought of my nephew Charlie's funeral, when the lady-bugs landed on his coffin. Of summer days. Of the little gift on my nightstand back home.

"That's good luck," Stephanie said. "That's a blessing."

"There's another one," Marina said, as we stepped off.

We were sixty-seven floors up in the middle of Manhattan, surrounded by ladybugs. A blessing.

Stephanie pushed me out onto the viewing balcony. From that height, New York City looked like Legoland, the millions of people hidden away. We were on top of the world.

I ask you now to set aside your opinion about same-sex marriage for these few minutes as you read. There was already a woman at the wedding—a relative of Pam's—who advertised her disapproval.

This is not about morals or the Bible. This is about Kerri, a friend for many years. An always-there-for-you type of person. Someone I saw struggle with relationships for years. A single mother who sacrificed for her children, who worked hard, but never found joy in her personal life.

Until she met Pam.

"This is it, Kerri," I had told her. "This is the joy you have been waiting for. And you deserve it."

She cried. "I know," she said, "and I almost gave up."

I wanted to be at the wedding for Marina. Because I won't be there when Marina marries, but I want her to know that whomever she chooses—man or woman, black, red, purple, or brown—I support her. As long as that person makes her happy and treats her well, I support her.

And I wanted to be there for Kerri.

She had given me a gift in the lobby. Just like Kerri—a

gift given, when one was meant to be received. While we waited for the brides, I opened it. It was a necklace etched with the word *Serendipity*. Kerri and Pam had adopted my word as their own.

I put on the necklace, alongside the pendant of Saint Andreas that Soulla had give me in Cyprus. The one Panos had in his pocket the day he died.

The brides walked out. Kerri's ice-blue dress lit up her blue eyes. Pam, for the first time I had seen, was without her scientist spectacles, revealing her large, gorgeous brown eyes.

I hoped they might glance past each other's faces at the city below. The millions of people in all those Lego towers. A reminder of the extraordinary blessing—the serendipity—of finding the one person among millions who lights your soul.

But Kerri and Pam already felt that.

You could hear it in their words. See it in the joy on their faces.

Feel it when the minister said, "I now pronounce you married," and Pam said, barely, through her tears, "I never thought I'd hear those words."

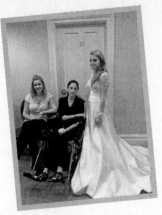

Kleinfeld's

The story of our trip to Kleinfeld's cannot be understood without further zooming into focus on this fourteen-year-old who is my daughter.

Key word there: *fourteen.*

On the plane to New York, Marina told me of a middle school band trip she had taken recently where a member of the band chewed up granola bars, spit them into a barf bag, and added orange juice for a true vomit effect. She thought that was hilarious.

As we pulled up to our hotel on Times Square, Marina noticed one of her favorite clothing stores across the street. "Oh my gosh! It's three stories!"

Inside the hotel one eve, we boarded an elevator with pizza boxes. Another couple in the elevator also had pizza, and we chatted pizza with them.

"Man, that was AWK-ward!" Marina said of the pizza chatter as we got off the elevator.

This was the girl I took to the fancy store for wedding dresses.

A child.

An awkward, beautiful child.

I'd arranged the visit with Kleinfeld's months in advance: sweating the details, assuaging the management, convincing the store they should allow us to come in for a special fitting even though we were not buying a dress.

As the trip approached, I would ask Marina if she was excited. "Yeah," she'd say in her high-pitched squeaky voice, the one she uses when she's really not sure.

"Sure, Mom," she'd say, shrugging her shoulders.

She still gushed about that tattoo parlor, though.

Yes, Marina was more enthused about (almost) getting a blue cornflower on her ankle to represent her mom's fight with ALS than trying on stinkin' $10,000 wedding gowns.

Awkward, beautiful, dear.

Friday morning was our Kleinfeld's visit. Stephanie and Marina arranged for a car service to take us the twenty-five blocks: an over-the-top handicapped van with a wheelchair lift, though I was able to get out of my wheelchair with assistance and transfer into a normal car.

The electric gates and ramps opened. The driver wheeled me in and strapped me down like Hannibal Lecter, then closed everything up.

"I feel like I'm taking you to the dog pound!" Steph said, cracking up.

I laughed too.

I knew if I started crying, I might never stop.

On the ride, Marina kept turning and looking at me in the back of the van. "You okay, Mom?"

"I am fine," I said.

At Kleinfeld's, I was unloaded like a piece of cargo. We rolled across the bustling, dirty city sidewalk—with scaffolding overhead and the distinct smell of marijuana—and into a dream.

Flower arrangements ten feet high. White grillwork on a Romeo-and-Juliet balcony. An ivory gown posed with a black tuxedo, a headless bride and groom.

"Wow!" I said.

I was wearing a new black outfit, one of four I had shopped for with Stephanie before the trip. Marina wore jean shorts, a sleeveless shirt, and sneakers. She stood with her hands crossed over her chest, looking like this was the last place on the planet she wanted to be.

Even "Remember that from the show?" drew little more than a nod.

The kind Kleinfeld ladies began walking us around the showroom. Stephanie pushed my chair, Marina beside me. They pointed out rooms like practiced tour guides, naming off the designers on display. Alita Graham. Pnina Tornai. There were rows and rows of dresses. Bedazzled. Be-blinged. Tulle clouds that made Princess Diana's dress look modest.

Marina said not a word.

We turned the corner to the dressing rooms. The white salon. The famous storage room where hundreds of dresses hang in plastic protector sleeves. The one Randy scurries back to on the show to pluck out "the One" for the flummoxed bridezilla fighting with her mother in the fitting room.

On television, the storage room is a smorgasbord of frosted delights. In real life, it's a glorified closet. That morning, Kleinfeld's seemed much smaller.

And the dresses much larger, like they were for eight-foot fairy-tale brides in castle weddings. The Spencer-Wendel women are barely over five feet tall.

Marina and I were overwhelmed.

"Want to try one on?" I slurred, touching Marina's hand. We were in a room full of flying dresses, looking up at their bottoms. Extra storage, we were told. A conveyor belt of dresses that stretched all the way to the next block.

"Okay," Marina said in her squeaky voice.

"Tell them the style you'd like. Pick a silhouette."

"Pick a silhouette" means pick the shape of the dress—wide ball gown, straight, A-line.

Marina stood mute.

I felt badly for bringing her. For foisting such an adult experience on a child. And crying, I knew, would only ramp that up a thousand times. So I held back.

As Marina disappeared silently into the dressing room, I tried not to think of my little girl on her wedding day.

I tried not to think of her as a baby in my arms. Nor her with her own baby in her arms one day.

I tried not to think of Marina right now, embarrassed by her mother's plans. By things she could not and should not yet understand.

Rather, I poured out wedding-dress tips to Stephanie.

I am leaving money in my will for Marina's wedding dress. Stephanie has promised to bring her back to Kleinfeld's to purchase it. Which in itself is crazy, amusing, and dear.

You see, Stephanie's all-time favorite clothing store is what we call the "Hoochie Mama" store, where tiny polyester sundresses and plastic stiletto shoes are all $9.99.

When we visited my publisher, I had to tell her, "Cover up. Wear something high on top." She often pours her ample chest into the polyester in such a way I worry about a wardrobe failure.

And this was the woman I was counting on to help Marina pick the most sophisticated and lavish dress of her life.

Alas. I just hoped the godawful glut of strapless gowns would be outsourced to China by then. In my opinion, they made women look like linebackers.

"No stark white!" I said to Stephanie. "Ivory. Not too much tulle. Think lace."

Marina had picked an A-line dress, one that flares out at the bottom like the letter. Or more precisely, the ladies of Kleinfeld's had picked it for her. Marina was too stunned to do more than nod.

"Think royalty when picking a dress," I counseled Steph, as we waited outside the dressing room. "Think Princess Kate. Sophisticated. Elegant. Think long sleeves. They transform dresses to more formal."

Marina came out.

Strapless. Flared. She looked like a fourteen-year-old girl parked in the middle of a giant cupcake, ready to tackle the quarterback.

"I don't like poofy," she said.

That's my girl!

"How 'bout trying on one with long sleeves?" I asked her.

I had mentioned to the Kleinfeld's folks that my all-time

favorite dress was the one Bella wore in the movie *Breaking Dawn*. A sheath of form-fitting silk with a sheer lace back and long sleeves with lace points extending over the hands.

The ladies brought out a dress similar to Bella's and Princess Kate's. Long lace sleeves and empire neckline, a ruched, fitted waist, long smooth silk skirt with a train.

Marina disappeared into the dressing room. I laid on "when the day comes" advice for Stephanie—"When the day comes, choose x." "When the day comes, do y." Advice I can't remember, for my heart was in that dressing room.

The door opened. Marina appeared, a foot taller and a decade older.

I could clearly see the beautiful woman she will be one day. I simply stared.

What do you do in bright-line moments, when your loss whomps you on the head? When you glimpse a moment you will not live to see?

I dipped my head. Breathe, I told myself.

I looked up. I smiled, and Marina smiled back. I worked my tongue into position to speak.

"I like it," I said.

Marina usually stands with a teenage hunch, but in that dress she stood straight, radiant and tall.

"You are beautiful," I whispered, my tongue barely co-operating. I don't know if she heard me. I was slurring and fighting tears.

We took some photos.

And moved on.

A memory made.

Marina returned the dress and went back to her jeans

shorts and sneakers. We rolled on quietly past the measuring room, the tuxedo room, the large underground room where dozens of women sat hunched over sewing machines.

There were too many people around to say what I wanted Marina to hear. How special she is to me.

That I will always be with her in spirit.

Always.

Kleinfeld's was not the place for such a conversation. Not with two saleswomen swirling around us, giving veil advice. Brides wandering red-eyed with team in tow. A stream of people cutting past us, ducking into changing rooms.

Kleinfeld's had been hesitant to let us try on dresses, worried that scads of terminally ill mothers might descend on them. No worries. Kleinfeld's was not the place for saying the words you hope your daughter will remember all her life.

Which probably is for the best.

For Marina is a child.

A child counting on her mother to be with her. To protect her.

They loaded me back into the handicap van, with its wheelchair cage. Steph made the same joke about the dog pound. I laughed to keep from crying. Oh sweet sister, don't break my heart.

"Can we get pizza on the way back?" was all Marina said.

"Of course," I replied.

That night as I slept, Marina lay down beside me.

"You are so cute, Mom," Stephanie heard her say.

She kissed me.

When I awoke the next morning, my daughter was sleeping beside me.

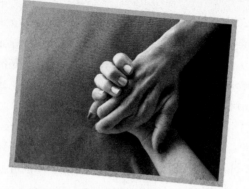

For Good

Our final night in New York, we made it a night just for the three of us: Marina, Stephanie, and me.

On the trip, there had been no discussions with Marina about illness or death. Not for a child who thinks small talk about pizza is awkward. Not for a child so thrilled by her new clothes bought in New York.

"It was on sale and the only extra small!" she squealed about a black miniskirt from the three-story wonder store by the hotel.

No, no deep discussions for her. What-oh-what would I even say?

So that final eve we did something where you don't have to talk. Something that left us speechless. We went to a Broadway show: *Wicked*.

It's a riff on *The Wizard of Oz*—the backstory of the friendship between Glinda the Good Witch and the green Wicked Witch. It was spectacular, with flying monkeys and gorgeous costumes and a green-skinned star who sang her heart out. I sat beside Marina. I touched her hand with my curled fingers, grateful for the dark silence and extravaganza before us.

In New York, I had cried once, when someone asked me to talk about my children. I didn't cry at Kleinfeld's, seeing Marina in that gown. Nor at the wedding. Nor when I was schlepped in that handicapped van like a piece of cargo.

Not until Marina leaned over to me in the dark theater and began singing along with the show, a song called "For Good." The witches were singing good-bye to one another, accompanied by harp and horn.

> *It well may be*
> *That we will never meet again*
> *In this lifetime,*

Marina softly sang.
My heart pounded, eyes welled.

> *So let me say before we part*
> *So much of me*
> *Is made of what I learned from you.*
> *You'll be with me*
> *Like a handprint on my heart.*

I looked at my girl. My little girl. Slowly, I raised my hand, and wiped away tears. Beside me, Marina wiped hers away as well.

When the show was over, I asked her why she was crying.

"Because you were, Mom."

Okay, I thought. No more of that.

Captiva
Island

August

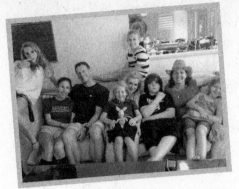

The Lion's Paw

My son Aubrey wanted to go to Sanibel Island, Florida, for his special trip. He had gone a few years before with our neighbor Sabra and her children, and it was his favorite place.

Sanibel Island, and its neighbor Captiva Island, are long, flat barrier islands off the west coast of Florida, places renowned for their seashells and sunsets.

Mind you, not all beaches have shells. The Florida beach I live near on the east coast usually has just a thin strip of inch-longers and broken fragments deposited by the tide. Sanibel and Captiva are positioned at such an angle to the Gulf of Mexico that millions of shells wash up on their shores.

A seeker's dream.

And the islands were only a three-hour drive west of Palm Beach, an easy jaunt across Florida's inland swamp. A close world, a familiar one, but separate and special nonetheless.

Wonderful, I thought. Perfect.

I set to work.

Aubrey and I sat in the Chickee hut and looked over websites. He chose a house on Captiva Island that slept ten, right next to the beach. It was three stories tall, "with an elevator, Mom, so you can go up and down."

We would be there for a week in late August, with John and the other kids, Nancy and her children, Steph and her family, cycling through. But the first three days would be for me and Aubrey.

And Steph, my caretaking companion.

I knew exactly the memory I wanted to plant.

As children, Steph and I had mooned over a book called *The Lion's Paw*. As soon as we read it—in fourth grade for both of us—it was our favorite book.

We loved Nick and Penny, a brother and sister who run away from a cruel orphanage in search of a better life. They meet Ben, a teenager whose father has gone missing in the war. Ben is convinced that if he finds a lion's paw, a rare shell found on and around Sanibel and Captiva, his lost father will return to him.

The children steal away on Ben's father's boat in search of that small shell. They travel all over south Florida, fighting alligators, hiding in mangroves, outwitting pursuers, forming a tight friendship, learning lessons, and having the adventures of a lifetime.

For years, I wanted to be like Penny or Nick or even Ben. I wanted to steal away and find what I was missing in my life.

I own a lion's paw shell, a fully intact one, with all five "knuckles." Knuckles are knobs on the shell that make it resemble a real animal paw. I received my shell as a young adult and kept it through children and travels and career, one of my prized possessions.

I love it because, on first glance, the lion's paw is not unique. It is the basic fan shape of almost every shell in the ocean, with a preponderance of brown.

But a true lion's paw comes from one particular species of scallop.

It is the size of a fist. The distinctive ridges are so high and curved they look almost like toes. And the color, on closer inspection, is not brown, but a dozen shades of orange, with purple bands that spiral and melt, or striate the shell, or mix with the orange into ochre. A glance-and-you-might-miss-it beauty, but one that grows the more you look. Each shell a story in itself.

I decided to take my lion's paw to Captiva.

After reading the book with Aubrey, I would take my old-soul son to the beach. One of the landing-strip-wide sections. We would talk of the story of the lion's paw as the sun set, painting the sky my favorite colors—sapphire, mango, magenta.

Then, "Oh, look, a lion's paw." My lion's paw, the edge poking out of the sand just where Stephanie buried it.

Aubrey would smile. He'd probably say, "Here, Mom. You keep it." But I'd say, "No, no, no, it's yours, my boy. You found it, just like Nick and Penny. Keep it all your life."

Eye-heart-u, son.

Eye-heart-u, too.

Of course, if you've read up to here, you know events rarely happen as anticipated. The no-show northern lights, Stephanie upchucking on the cruise, Panos's Bible, even Kleinfeld's—none of those things turned out just as planned.

But were perfect memories, nonetheless.

Because I did not have expectations. I guess that's a lesson, if there must be one. Accept the life that comes. Work and strive, but accept. Don't force the world to be the one you dream.

The reality is better.

So I did not fret when a host of things went wrong with the Aubrey plan.

"Your mom tells me she has a lion's paw!" Ellen said to Aubrey. Ugh. Capsize the surprise, why don't you?

My parents told some friends, who kindly bought a lion's paw online. My mother gave it to Aubrey with such glee. It wasn't a real lion's paw, but Aubrey thought it was. Sheeeeesh!

And of course Aubrey wasn't eager to read the book.

Steph chased him around the house for half the summer: "Sugarplum, don't ya wanna read? It's my favorite book! And it's about Sanibel!"

"No," he'd say.

I decided to read it with Aubrey. But my voice was too slurred, and he had no interest in sitting down and reading to his mom.

No bother.

The real problem hit the moment we arrived at our house on Captiva Island. The beach. I had begun to form the plan four months before. Back then, I could have walked out with Aubrey. Not far, but far enough.

But now, after the exhaustion of Cyprus and New York, and four more months of ALS, I could not walk unassisted. Especially on loose sand.

Do not pine for things you cannot have, I thought, for that is the way to the loony bin.

I turned away. Went inside our rented house, furnished just so, with a screened pool and jacuzzi, private balconies, five bedrooms, a spiral staircase, a house so lavish and nice that Aubrey didn't want to leave.

"There's a flat-screen TV in every bedroom!" Aubrey gushed.

He was knee-deep in a two-pound tub of Jelly Belly jelly beans. Jelly Bellies come in scads of flavors, like buttered popcorn, cotton candy, cappuccino, and plum. Aubrey would fish out two matching beans for Steph and me, and we'd guess the flavor. He manned the flavor guide.

"No! No! That was pomegranate!" he'd say.

Here's Aubrey in a nutshell: the other night, he expressed concern about John going back to college soon. "Dad, you're gonna get pantsed. The younger students will tease you and pull your pants down."

When Aubrey gained admission to a prestigious arts middle school this year, he declined to tell a buddy in his band who hadn't made it. He didn't want to hurt her feelings.

Aubrey enjoyed quiet moments with me. But three days? I knew he would enjoy company more. So I invited Nancy and her children, Liam and Devin, who met us there.

"There's an elevator!" sunny Devin announced. "In a house!"

"Yes, dear, it's for Susan," said Nancy.

Now this elevator would be a blessing and a curse. Because at each story it had two doors that had to be closed tightly for it to operate, and these doors tended to stick.

The elevator was the size of a closet, fitting a wheelchair and two people at most. And it was so stuffy inside, the house caretaker asked us to keep the doors open to air it out. There was no emergency phone or alarm, just a lone wire. If the doors got stuck, which they often did, you poked a metal rod in a hole above the door and it was supposed to pop open. Supposed to.

Of course, the doors immediately stuck. Wouldn't open to let me in. Nancy and Steph ran up and down the stairs, ensuring all the doors were closed so the elevator would operate.

Finally, they had to carry me up the stairs.

Steph grabbed me under the armpits, and Nancy grabbed my feet. Imagine a ninety-five-pound sack of potatoes. Now schlep it up two flights of stairs.

Nancy, bearing my lighter end, wanted to move quickly. Steph with the heavier end: NOT. They kept plopping me on my bum, as gently as they could, but not as gently as I liked.

Ergo, I was happy to stay on my third-floor private balcony, writing, enjoying the rustle of the palm tree beside me. The balcony became my command center. My place to be alone, a state I was becoming more and more comfortable with.

I sat on my balcony while the kids explored the house. Turned on every television. Went to the beach with Nancy and Steph. Polished off the entire two-pound container of Jelly Bellies.

I was not imposing myself on Aubrey. Not forcing him to be near me. He was close. He was having fun, and that was enough.

In the evening, I came down to lounge. We marinated and grilled steaks, since Aubrey loves steak. Nancy nearly ignited herself along with the gas grill.

Over dinner, we played Table Topics, a game we found in the house. Cards with questions you can talk about: "If you could meet one famous person, who would it be?" Barack Obama. "Do you love the beach or mountains more?" The beach, of course. (Steph and I resolved to get the game and play it with our parents, to try to get to know them better.) One question for everyone: "When you die, where do you want your remains put?"

And my old-soul son said: "At the graves of my parents."

The game moved on. The kids went for ice cream.

Alone in bed, I cried myself to sleep.

"Come on, sugarplums! Let's read!" I heard Stephanie calling the next morning. She was reading *The Lion's Paw* to the kids at every opportunity. Nancy's children, Liam and Devin, were interested. Aubrey was becoming so.

I texted John. "Come on over," I told him. If it was a party, I wanted everyone there.

That morning, Nancy's sister Sally and her husband Paul took us boating. I have been crestfallen when friends who used to invite me boating no longer do so. We sat in the back of the boat, chatting, sunning, enjoying the salt air. Flying over the water, but feeling still. Sally and Paul made my day, and Aubrey's too.

John arrived with Wesley, Marina, and Marina's friend Lizzy. The tenor of the house began to change. Aubrey and Marina argued. Marina disappeared as often as she could with Lizzy. Wesley drove a golf cart (came with the house) into the garage wall.

I stayed on my balcony, above the chaos. Letting the

noises swirl up to me. Occasionally a child with a question. Or Aubrey, trying to get away from Wes. Or an adult came around to sit with me or ask if I was all right.

I got my Zen on. Tapped out this book, writing the chapter on the space shuttle. Watching the clouds blow across the sky.

"What would I do without this book?" I asked Steph at one point.

Because without it, I would have wanted to be down there with my children, with my friends, and wanting is the hardest part.

One afternoon, I lay down to rest. John helped me into the king-size bed, turned me on my hip, positioned me just the way I like. I love to have a pillow between my legs, so my bones don't hit together, and I hate to have hair over the ear against the pillow. These are the little things John knows, the little details he always takes care of, because finding the comfy spot, for me, is bliss.

I was lying there all snuggled on down comforters when I heard Wesley's muffled voice: "Help! Help!"

Silence. He screamed again.

"Help!"

I listened for a response downstairs. I heard someone yell: "Oh, no! Wes is stuck in the elevator!"

I tried to roll over. To get to him.

Oh boy, I thought. I hope they find that metal rod. And I hope it works.

Wesley continued calling out: "I'm stuck! I'm stuck!" His voice was rising.

I heard people far away: "It's okay, baby. We're getting you out."

I waited, stuck and alone. Listening so intently I could have heard an atom move.

And then Wesley started wailing like I've never heard before. Wailing like a wild animal shot. He was hysterical.

I thought of him trapped inside the stuffy elevator alone, gulping down the finite amount of oxygen in there.

I tried again to inch myself to the edge of the bed, intent on flinging myself to the floor and crawling out of the bedroom.

Wes wailed and wailed, louder and louder. It seemed to go on and on.

I imagined him red and sweating, his blue eyes bulging in terror. I imagined those elevator walls closing in on him.

Why aren't they calling the fire department? I thought.

I had no phone. I couldn't move. I couldn't help my son.

I had a panic attack and began wailing. "Help! Help!" I yelled as loud as I could, which isn't very loud.

Finally John rushed into the bedroom to find me slumped against the side of the bed. I had managed to slide myself off the mattress onto the floor, but I couldn't stand up. "What happened?" John said. "Susan, what's wrong?"

"Call fucking nine-one-one!"

"Why?"

"Because your goddamned son is stuck in an elevator!"

"He's out! He's out!" John said. "He's crying because it scared him."

"Are you sure? Are you lying?"

"No. He's fine. Hysterical, but fine."

Stephanie later described for me how Wesley threw himself on chairs—"flopping round like a trout," as she put it—

after being released from the elevator. "He was calmer stuck inside," Steph said.

Again, that night, I cried myself to sleep.

Steph's family joined us for the last few days in Captiva. Husband Don, sons William and Stephen, and their girlfriends, Kristi and Kami. The days grew long and lazy. Lounging, swimming, eating, laughing, just being together.

Steph's boys, always so affectionate with their mom, were openly affectionate with their girlfriends in front of her. Which was so dear to see. John and I have been married twenty years, yet I would still feel odd snugglin' with him in front of my parents.

Aubrey relished the fact we had gathered for him. I heard him say to another child: "You know, this is MY vacation."

He said it not in a haughty way, but in a happy way.

"You know how this is my trip?" he said to me near the end. "Well, there's something I really want to do."

I bet it's not find a lion's paw, I thought.

"I'd like to go parasailing," he said.

He had seen people parasailing on the beach. An activity where you essentially strap into a sail behind a boat, and the boat speeds along, lifting you thirty, forty feet aloft in flight.

Mind you, Aubrey is eleven.

"How old do you have to be?" I asked, thinking surely they don't allow children to do such a hazardous thing.

"Just six years old!" Aubrey said, beaming. "They take kids as young as six."

"Ah! Don't say a word to your brother!"

Aubrey is a small human being, like me, often turned

away at rides by height requirements. He's still smarting from his last trip to Sea World, where he was half an inch too short for the roller coasters.

"Is there a height requirement?" I asked, halfway hoping there might be one.

"No!" Aubrey said, thrilled.

Now, Aubrey is no daredevil child. If he was eager to do it, who was I to stop him? Let him try new things, I told myself. Let him experience life. Parasail. Eat chile peppers. Jump off short bridges. Don't fear the alligator in the canal if you do not see it there. Fearing the possible is no way to live.

Aubrey rode in tandem with his cousin, Will, eighteen. I did not go to watch, not wanting the rigamarole of moving me around to detract from his experience. I couldn't see him from my balcony, but I could imagine him out there, flying free, laughing.

I liked the idea of Aubrey out there, soaring without me.

He loved it. For twelve whole minutes, he sailed above the shore. "So high! The people on the beach, they looked about this big," he said, holding his thumb and forefinger about an inch apart.

"Ack! Were you scared?"

"No. Well . . . yes, at first. I was petrified."

Then cousin Will adjusted him, and he realized the harness would hold, and Aubrey relaxed.

And looked around in wonder.

At the green water along the beach, which melded to blue farther offshore. At the smooth dunes in the distance. At the tiny figures on the sand.

And he listened to silence.

"It was so quiet!" Aubrey said. There was just one errant flap on the sail, slapped repeatedly by the wind.

"It was silent except for that," Aubrey said. "It was so cool!"

In the end, there was no chance for a quiet moment to sit with Aubrey. No chance to present Aubrey with my lion's paw. The final chapters of the book we left unread.

It was for the best. The shell, I realized, was an awful gift for Aubrey. I was so focused on my Hollywood moment with him that I forgot what the shell represents in the book: that if you are lucky enough to have one, your parent will return.

I will not return to Aubrey, at least not in the flesh.

But I will, I hope, in spirit. In the things he sees and feels. In the memories we made.

Look for me in your heart, my children. Sense me there, and smile, just as I sensed Panos in that decrepit monastery.

Look for me in the sunset.

All their lives, I have marveled in front of my children at sunsets. "Isn't it gorgeous?" I've gushed.

Now they do the same.

"Look!" said Aubrey recently of clouds glowing gold and pink and orange.

Marina talks of wanting to live in New York City one day. Wesley of being a dolphin trainer, or caring for sea turtles. Their memories already abloom.

I am not gone. I have today. I have more to give.

I know the end is coming, but I do not despair.

I have complete peace that my children will be well cared

for. That John, Stephanie, and Nancy will tend their gardens and their souls.

They have promised to take Aubrey to Cyprus to meet his relatives, the ones he looks so much like. They have promised to help Marina with her wedding dress. They have promised to foster Wesley's remarkable drawing talents.

I leave you, my children, the memories of all we enjoyed and discovered.

I leave this book. The one I worked on each day for most of our magical year. Tap, tap, tapping with my last finger, one letter at a time.

M-A-R-I-N-A

A-U-B-R-E-Y

W-E-S-L-E-Y

G-O-O-D-B-Y-E my loves.

Afterword

October 2013

Editor's Note

We asked Susan if she wanted to submit anything new for the paperback edition of her book. She was in at-home hospice and had lost the ability to speak and type, so we did not expect anything. A week later, she submitted the following, written with the help of a HeadMouse, a camera that reads a reflective dot on her nose, allowing her to type. Here's what she and "Dotty" wrote.

Living Things

Life, inexorable, surges on.

I can no longer walk or talk or eat well. But the children's lives continue, as normal as possible, as they should.

They're full of friends, activities, concerts, and concerns about academics, fashion, and changing bodies—all the travails of childhood.

They don't ask about my future; they ask about the weekend's activities.

I think of flowers. Cause, ya know: "Earth laughs in flowers." (Ralph Waldo Emerson wrote that in a poem.)

And, boy, we need brightness and laughter.

Soon after the book was finished, I discovered that the South Florida School of Floral Design, founded in 1963, was right near my house.

"Would you take me to flower school? And be my hands?" I asked John.

"Are you serious?" he said.

We called the school, and an older-sounding man named Walter answered. We explained the "situation," that I could not use my hands but that my husband would arrange the flowers for me.

"I'll alert the Marine band of your arrival!" Walter said.

What a wiseass, I thought.

The class was at 7:30 a.m. We arrived late, as always. John rolled me over the front stoop . . . and back in time. There were linoleum high-top counters and vintage wooden desks, the armchair tablet kind I had in elementary school. A few were set out in front of a large blackboard; a dozen more were piled up, unused.

There was a little sign on the blackboard that read: "Martha Stewart doesn't live here, and it's a good thing."

Know those flower arrangements that are beautiful in their simplicity? Walter's voice drips derision as he says their name: "Roundy moundies." Martha Stewart, he says, made them popular and sapped the artistry out of floral arranging.

Well, I love nice modern roundy moundies. I began to doubt that Walter's course was the right one for me.

But then Walter began teaching. And in between lessons on how to make fresh-cut flowers last longer and how to tie a gorgeous bow, Walter, seventy-eight years young, told of himself.

He and his wife had six children. She had died years ago, after forty-one years of marriage. One of their sons had died at age twelve, and another son was soon to be sent to prison for murder.

Walter had worked for twenty years as a volunteer at a hospice and had seen more than life's fair share of sorrow.

But teaching in front of the class, arranging flowers, he was happy. He was at home.

After we left class, Walter wrote wise letters to John and me, about what he had learned of life and death. He wrote that John and I had helped him heal from his son's death thirty-seven years ago.

Hearing that made me so happy, I cried for a half hour.

Since I began this fast track to death, deeper souls like Walter seem drawn to me.

Walter said he'd do anything he could to help us. So when Stephanie's son, Stephen, had his senior prom, I volunteered Walter to make the corsage and boutonniere. I advised Stephanie that Walter tends to make them way too large. I mean, seven flowers in a corsage? Crazy!

"Let's tell him they're midgets," I told Steph.

Walter was thrilled to help. "I'll notify the Marine band you're coming," he said.

What a dear man, I thought.

After my book was published, I began to hear from soulful readers across continents.

Hello from Iowa, Manitoba, China! Blessings from Mexico and Finland. Salutations from Sri Lanka. Best wishes from Washington.

Many, many readers wrote that the book inspired them. This delights every cell of my being. It gives me the feeling that I have left a positive charge out there in the world.

Of course, there were struggles. There always are.

A major one for me was a few people who withdrew from me. People who were intensely close to me for at least a third of my life.

But the day I was diagnosed with ALS, it was as if our relationships were irradiated. And slowly they died.

These people asked for a free copy of my book, then said nothing to me that indicated they even read it.

I asked one if he'd like me to write something personal for him. (It was the only thing I could do anymore.) "No" was the instant answer.

Then the window of opportunity to speak final words with these folks slammed shut. I lost my voice.

I asked them to come and read to me, no conversation required, hoping to give them a reason to come and sit near me. That, too, was a fail. I realized they were uncomfortable with a muted me.

I was furious. I daydreamed about how I could hurt them as much as they'd hurt me.

But what would that accomplish? Only engender more bitterness and prove me an ass as well.

No thanks.

Leave a positive charge.

I thought often of the American Indian saying about how there are two wolves at odds within each of us. One wolf is angry, vengeful, arrogant. The other is serene, forgiving, humble.

The one who wins is the one you feed.

I quit feeding Facebook to the bad wolf. (Oh look! They went fishing instead of helping me.)

I fed the good wolf an aphorism instead: Focus not on people who let you down, but on those who lift you up.

It must be more than a thousand times now that John Wendel has lifted me up.

He wraps his six-and-a-half-foot span of arms around me and lifts me from the bed to the toilet to the wheelchair to the sofa and back again. Again, again, and again.

John hoists me as if he's hugging me. But I am dead weight, unable to support myself or hold on to him at all. John has developed tendonitis in his elbows and has wrenched his back a number of times. He continues to lift me without fail.

It certainly puts in perspective the many times during our twenty-two years of marriage that I chafed at John's lack of romanticism and thought, "He doesn't love me well enough."

Truth be told, John Wendel is a host of wonderful things. He is good-natured, loyal, industrious, fun, and handsome. But he isn't a whit romantic.

He doesn't pine away, send flowers, or plan delightful getaways for anyone.

For one anniversary, we went away for an evening. I managed to pour myself into a slinky strapless red dress, which, after birthing and nursing three children, was no small feat. (With the help of specially selected scaffolding, the dress looked nice.)

At dinner, John stared at other women. Then he took me to a nearby hotel where he had made our reservation. Except it wasn't a hotel: it was a flophouse, for rent by the hour, night, or month. "The lobby didn't look that bad!" John said in his own defense.

If I hadn't known better, I might have thought John was dissing me big time. But he was just being John.

John—LOUSY at the niceties of love.

John—OUTSTANDING at the essence of love.

Again and again and again.

There's a cast of characters, really, who lift me up. And John, too. They lift US up.

There's a man named Steve Sylvester. Before I got sick, I'd see Steve at a party now and again. All I knew of him was: 1) he was a physical therapist and 2) he liked Bud Light.

One thing that really sucks about being an ALS patient in hospice care is that physical therapy is not covered. We ALS patients must sit around while our muscles shrivel.

Steve offered to continue treating me after my insurance stopped paying for physical therapy. I pay him beans, and he works me over. My hamstrings feel as if they are going to snap in half—it hurts so damn good. And afterward, I stand better. I feel better.

An acquaintance from high school offered to massage me. For years, Liz Camp Nowacki has given me an hour of silent delight each week.

Then there's my best foodie friend, Tory Malmer. We brainstorm gourmet goop I can still swallow. She often texts me: "I'll be happy to make anything you crave."

"Let's make something with culinary lavender," I text, and get a smiley face in return.

My friend Jane Victoria Smith organized a passel of people who walked in ALS events and raised money for a cure.

Steve, Liz, Tory, Jane all surprised me with their goodness.

No surprise at all is the soul of my sister, Stephanie.

She comes to see me every day after her long day of work. "Helloooooo!" she sings as she steps in the door.

It's my favorite part of the day.

I lay on the sofa as Steph sits with my feet in her lap. Steph rubs my feet for hours, kneads and kneads the swelling. She presses her thumbs in the center of my sole, then walks them up and down. Heaven!

In this quiet, our minds meld.

"I'm okay with everything," I try to tell her. Somehow she understands.

"If you're okay, I'm okay," she says.

"My right shoe is bothering me."

She immediately bends down and undoes my left shoe.

We laugh and laugh, as Steph does this every time.

She's an extraordinary health-care provider. I see this when she feeds me. Steph's so patient and instinctive. She knows when to offer a sip of soda, when to wait, when to wipe, and what to do when someone chokes.

She doesn't stand there screaming, "Oh my gawd!!!!" and ratcheting my panic up to DEFCON 5.

Rather, she quietly asks me while I'm turning blue, "Are you moving air?" "Do you want me to call 911?" or "Do you want me to shut up?"

To help John, Steph will sometimes spend the night, giving him a break from turning me in bed every few hours. I look forward to those nights like a child looks forward to a

sleepover. As children, we were rarely allowed to sleep together.

Stephanie and Susan. Made sisters by forces unknown.
Positively charged forces.

Stephanie is an empty-nester now, her sons just off to college. And I am unable to move or speak to my children. This
timing is a blessing.

Our time together is enjoyable and peaceful. We're okay.

Until Wesley acts out.

Yesterday, he came into the room and spit water in our
general direction. Wes was pissed that John had picked him
up from school and not his second-favorite person in the
world, Yvette.

Wes gets upset when routines are broken. Routine is central to autistic children.

Wesley behaves, though, when Steph tells him she will
leave if he continues spitting, hitting, or whatever.

'Cause Steph is his number-one favorite person.

The only one he'll hug as he falls asleep.

He is clearly bonded with her now, as all of the children are.

Aubrey knows that if he looks at Steph a certain way she'll
take him to buy candy.

Marina, a sophomore in high school, is finally focused on
college plans. She talks often about them with Stephanie.

Marina said to me the other day: "You know, Steph laughs
at everything. It's so great."

I nodded my head emphatically: yes.

In floral school, John learned how to turn a dozen daisies,
violet statice, and leatherleaf greenery into a big spray ar-

rangement you can sell for $50. Walter proclaimed him a "good" floral designer.

John said he enjoyed the quiet concentration of creating with living things.

As part of the class, we visited a nursery and overlooked rows of billowing green. The Easter lilies were growing precisely in time for their March 31 delivery, their baby buds just beginning to peer up.

"I love being outside," John said that day.

Not long after, John set his sights on a new career—as a farmer.

John had read about a new method of farming called aquaponics. It's a method in which you grow food plants in conjunction with fish tanks.

Huh?

That's what I said, too.

John launched into a lecture about how the fish fertilize the plants growing in the water. He was thrilled with the idea. He began growing his hair long again so he would look like an organic farmer. He talked of growing gourmet minigreens and vegetables. He went to aquaponics school.

Normally, I'd be ringin' every alarm bell possible about profitability and feasibility. "John," I'd usually ask with unfettered incredulity, "how will you fare in the gourmet games when you believe that all humans really need to eat is sweet potatoes?"

(He once ate so many sweet potatoes his palms turned orange.)

But I said not a word.

"Perfect," I thought. "It's a fresh life for John. One he is eager for."

John, enthused. Children, bonded. All well provided for.

Content, I'd press the Exit-Earth-Now button if I had one. And sidestep the only thing left to do.

Ah, if we could just disappear—poof!

Then write upon a luminous moon, like icing on a cake: "Keep Calm & Carry On. Love you, Mom."

Don't cry because it's over.
Smile because it happened.

—DR. SEUSS

Acknowledgments

In addition to those named in this book, I would like to thank the invisible people.

The ones who opened worlds for me.

For example, my teachers who inspired learning. I had outstanding ones, including Mrs. Herpel, Mr. Signer, Mr. Trotsky, and UNC professor Dr. Andrew Scott, who helped me land an internship at the United Nations, forever altering my worldview.

And my colleagues at the *Palm Beach Post*, who encouraged me as a writer, investigator, experience seeker.

My sincere thanks go to my coauthor, Bret Witter, who kept rearranging the furniture in the book until it felt right.

And to my agent, Peter McGuigan of Foundry Literary, who took a chance on me, a writer who could no longer type. Wow!

Also of Foundry, Stephanie Abou, Rachel Hecht, and Matt Wise.

HarperCollins editor Claire Wachtel's flinty evaluation elevated the book.

Also at HarperCollins, Rachel Elinsky, Tina Andreadis, Leah Wasielewski, and Jonathan Burnham.

Beyond my every fantasy, Universal Pictures bought rights and may make a movie of this book. My thanks to agent Brandy Rivers, and to producers Scott Stuber and Alexa Faigen.

It is my hope that all those who profit from this story will donate to ALS research.

And you, kind reader, as well.

When I was a child, my mother, Tee, used to stand over me, insisting on better writing. She encouraged as well as criticized.

I acknowledge that no mother knows her child will write a book.

Thank you, Mom.

Photo Credits

Photo on page 35 by Gary Coronado, *Palm Beach Post*

Photo on page 111 by Moya Photography

Photo on page 123 by Moya Photography

Photo on page 141 by Greg Lovett, *Palm Beach Post*

Photo on page 222 by Greg Lovett, *Palm Beach Post*

All others courtesy of the author and her family

About the Author

Susan Spencer-Wendel was an award-winning journalist at the *Palm Beach Post* for almost twenty years. A graduate of the University of North Carolina at Chapel Hill, she holds a master's degree in journalism from the University of Florida. She has been honored for her work by the Society of Professional Journalists and the Florida Press Club, and she received a lifetime achievement award for her court reporting from the Florida Bar. She lives in West Palm Beach, Florida, with her family.
www.susanspencerwendel.com

Bret Witter has collaborated on six *New York Times* bestsellers. He lives in Decatur, Georgia.
www.bretwitter.com